Motivate Healthy Habits:

Change yourself before helping others

Rick Botelho
Family Doctor

www.MotivateHealthyHabits.com

PREFACE

As a British-trained general practitioner who has been teaching family medicine in the United States for over 18 years, I have learned a great deal from patients, students, and health care practitioners, as well as from the research evidence and from different theories and models about health behavior change. In order to help in the training of health care professionals, I have written a two-part book series (*Beyond Advice: 1. Becoming a Motivational Practitioner and 2. Developing Motivational Skills*) that goes beyond current research evidence and incorporates state-of-the-art practices. To assist the general public, I have written this guidebook based on the above-mentioned work to help you (and others) on an inner journey of self-directed change.

Far more resources are invested in treating diseases than in changing unhealthy habits. Yet unhealthy habits account for half of all preventable deaths and 70% of all preventable costs in health care. Even with more resources devoted to promoting healthy habits, the size of this problem is still too big for the health care system, which simply cannot help everyone who has an unhealthy habit. Therefore, self-help and mutual help approaches are the first step in addressing this issue.

This book taps into the most important resource by mobilizing you, your family and friends to work on your own health behaviors. You may or may not need additional help. For this reason, this book will have a Web site where you and health care professionals can share and learn from one another about motivating healthy habits.

I hope you find this book useful in helping you change an unhealthy habit. Such learning can then help you become a better coach to help others you care about.

Visit **www.MotivateHealthyHabits.com**
to learn more, get more support, to buy books for friends and family members, listen to audio, watch videos, or read book outlines for health care professionals. For wholesale prices for book stores and Web sites, or bulk buys for health and training organizations, send an email to the address below.

© 2000 Richard J. Botelho, M.D.
Associate Professor of Family Medicine, Psychiatry and Nursing
Family Medicine Center, 885 South Avenue
Rochester, NY 14620-2399
Phone: (716) 442-7470, Ext. 508
Send suggestions for improvement to:
Rick_Botelho@Urmc.Rochester.Edu

To Eve, Anna, and Sara with love

Acknowledgments:

I would like to thank Peg Toohey, Marlene Mussell and Ceil Goldman for their editorial support, Steve Marcus for his secretarial support, Donald Botelho for his supportive critique, and my patients, students and professional colleagues who contributed in countless different ways over many years.

The major influences that have shaped the development of this guidebook and the 2-part practitioner book series are: the Transtheoretical Model of Change (Jim Prochaska and Carlos DiClemente), Motivational Interviewing (William Miller and Steve Rollnick), Self-Determination Theory (Ed Deci and Rich Ryan), Self-Efficacy Theory (Albert Bandura), Relapse Prevention (Allan Marlatt), and Solution-based Therapy (Steve De Shazer). These books build on the shoulders of these cutting-edge theorists, researchers and/or clinicians.

Motivate Healthy Habits:
Change yourself before helping others

Table of Contents

INTRODUCTION

Are you concerned about a family member or friend who has an unhealthy habit? What about you? Do you have any unhealthy habits? There is probably something that you can do to improve your own health. But often it is far easier to see what others need to do than to see what you need to do for yourself. So ask yourself this question: How can you help someone else change if you still need to change yourself?

KEY PRINCIPLE:

Put

Your

Health

First

Remember, being healthy involves caring about yourself as well as giving to others. If you are healthier, you are in a stronger position to give more, and help others change their unhealthy habits.

To put your health first is easier said than done though. This is because you have to do "inner change." Inner change goes beyond understanding your thoughts and feelings about your unhealthy habits. To work at inner change, you need to better understand and change your views and values as well.

EXPLORING INNER CHANGE

Let's begin with an everyday example of someone who used this guidebook, without help from others, to change an unhealthy habit. By comparing this person with an example of someone who had great difficulties in changing, you will learn more about inner change. Take note of your reactions as you read their stories. In spite of their differences, what is the common link between them?

An Everyday Example

Fred smoked nearly two packs of cigarettes a day. He regarded smoking cigarettes as his pacifier, but wanted to quit. He filled in a decision balance (see below) to help him explore his reasons to smoke versus his reasons to quit. (Chapters 3-5 will go into more detail on how to use the decision balance to work on inner change.)

Decision Balance

Choice A: To smoke	Choice B: To quit
Benefits of smoking *My pacifier.* *Relieves tension and anger.* *Something to do when not doing anything.* *Something to do when I am doing something.*	*Concerns about smoking* *Deadly pacifier.* *Health problems.* *Secondhand smoke for my family.* *Be an outcast and excluded.*
Concerns about quitting *Am I strong enough?* *How will I occupy my spare time?* *Will I need a new crutch?* *Will I have difficulties in concentrating?*	*Benefits of not smoking* *Taste food.* *Smell the air.* *Save money over time.* *Gain stamina.*
Reasons to smoke score (resistance) *Think score = 5 Feeling score = 10*	***Reasons to quit score (motivation)*** *Think score = 10 Feeling score = 10*

After completing a decision balance, Fred used a 0-10 scale (0 meaning "not important" and 10 meaning "very important") to rate what he thought and felt about his:
1. Reasons to stay the same (resistance score)
2. Reasons to change (motivation score)

On first reading this decision balance, you may have some difficulties in understanding the difference between thought and feeling scores about change. When you do this same exercise on yourself (see pp. 39-41), you will come to understand more directly, and see the importance of the difference. For example, your feelings are often a more potent driver of your behavior than your thoughts. You think you should change, but don't feel like it; you eat what you like, but know that you should stick to your diet. The scoring process can help you understand how your views about how you think and feel about change can vary and identify what influences your change in views over time. The challenge is how can you become truly passionate about putting your health first. The following example illustrates how Fred became passionate about quitting smoking.

Fred gave himself a resistance score of 5 and a motivation score of 10 based on what he thought about continuing to smoke and quitting. After admitting to himself that he felt hopeless about overcoming his nicotine addiction, he gave a resistance score of 10 and a motivation score of 10 based on what he felt. When Fred looked over his scores, he discovered how much he hated his nicotine addiction. He also discovered that he had strong mixed feelings about whether to quit or not, and felt he lacked the confidence to quit without additional help.

As Fred went through this book getting ready for change, he remembered how his parents had bought him candy cigarettes as a child. He discovered to his horror that candy cigarettes were still available in stores in his poor neighborhood. He also noticed that not only were they cheap (15 cents a pack), but that they were displayed in the stores at the height of small children, well below the sight line of parents. He was especially concerned, because he had two young children of his own. When he visited suburban supermarkets and discovered that candy cigarettes were not for sale in middle-class neighborhoods, he was so enraged that he decided to do something. He worked with his local church to begin community action against the neighborhood stores.

This guidebook helped Fred build up his confidence. He read through it to set a quit date and to use the nicotine patch. As a constant reminder not to smoke, he kept his book in the kitchen near the refrigerator, where he used to smoke cigarettes frequently. He came to use his book as his pacifier instead of cigarettes. He also used the nicotine patch with his quit-smoking attempts. Six months later, after his third quit attempt, he stopped smoking cigarettes for good.

A "Difficult to Change" Example

Mary had not used any safe sex practices for two years, even though her husband had human immunodeficiency virus (HIV). Her physician, who had just tested her and confirmed she was still HIV negative, informed her that it was just a matter of time before she got the virus. He asked her to fill out a decision balance (see below) to try and help her and him understand why she didn't want to protect herself.

Decision Balance

Choice A: Not to use condoms	Choice B: To use condoms every time
Benefits of not using condoms *Doesn't make him feel that he is sexually incompetent.* *He feels secure that I'll stay with him.*	*Concerns about not using condoms* *Don't want to get AIDS.* *Don't want my family hurt.* *Don't want people to think he doesn't care about protecting me.*
Concerns about using condoms every time *He will have erection problems and it will make him sad.* *He will wish he were with his ex-girlfriend (who is HIV positive) so he won't have to use them.*	*Benefits of using condoms every time* *Won't get HIV so I won't upset my family.* *Won't get sick myself so I can take care of him when he gets sick.* *Will feel that he cares enough about me so I do not get sick.*
Reasons to stay the same (resistance) *Think score = 6 Feeling score = 9*	***Reasons to change (motivation)*** *Think score = 8 Feeling score = 4*

Mary thought she should use condoms but her emotional reasons to stay the same were twice as important as her reasons to change. She was willing to sacrifice her life for her husband. When Mary's physician asked her to invite her husband to her next appointment, he attended one appointment. Two months later, she and her husband had relationship problems. Her physician then asked her to do another decision balance about whether she should stay in the relationship or separate from her husband. She wanted to stay with him, but he decided to separate. After the separation, she started to drink a lot of alcohol, after stopping for 10 years. Her physician suggested that she go to a treatment program for her alcohol problem. She did not want to go because she wanted to drown her sorrows. She said she would stop drinking when she got over him. Six months later, she stopped drinking alcohol without professional help.

Questions to think about:
What are the underlying reasons for why this woman put her life at risk?
How does this example make you feel toward Mary and her husband?
What are your thoughts and opinions about Mary and her husband?

The Common Factor Between These Two Examples

Both Fred and Mary sacrificed their long-term physical health for short-term emotional benefits. Fred sacrificed his physical health to benefit his own psychological well-being. In other words, he originally valued his short-term psychological health more than his long-term physical health. In contrast, Mary sacrificed her physical health for the psychological well-being of another person, her husband. By understanding what motivated them to act the way they did, it becomes easier for these individuals to work on inner change.

Now think about one of your unhealthy habits. In what ways are you sacrificing your long-term physical health for short-term psychological well-being?

BEGIN WITH YOURSELF

With advances in medical technology, health care systems will have to address the widening gap between the needs of people and the capacity to treat their diseases. Yet most of the preventable costs in health care are due to lifestyle behaviors: for example, tobacco is the leading cause of death internationally, and will remain so for the foreseeable future. Even though people know that smoking causes diseases, at least a quarter of the adult population still smokes, and youth smoking is on the increase. The smoking rates among the poor are unchanged in the United States, in spite of a decline in the overall smoking rate in the general population. Also, most people do not know that a quarter of all those who drink alcohol are at risk because they drink too much. Furthermore, lack of exercise and being overweight are common problems. Clearly, health care systems need to avoid such unnecessary costs in order to treat diseases more effectively. But health care systems do not have the capacity to treat all addictions (e.g., nicotine, alcohol, and drugs), let alone other unhealthy behaviors.

Health care planners talk about making individuals more responsible for leading healthier lifestyles. For example, they suggest giving incentives for healthy lifestyles, or charging higher health insurance rates to people with unhealthy habits. Giving rewards and punishments are simple ideas. But these ideas will not help the vast majority of people, because this approach does not address the need for change, at either an individual or societal level.

Health care systems alone cannot cope with or even address the magnitude of unhealthy behaviors. This is because we live in a disease-producing rather than a health-promoting society. Some of the greatest untapped resources for changing this situation are concerned family members, lay health organizations, such as Alcoholics Anonymous, and the Internet. In health-promoting societies, private and public sectors such as schools, community organizations, and the workplace will provide a wide range of effective resources for concerned family members. Together, they can help develop lay health organizations and use the World Wide Web to promote health. But you cannot wait until we get there. So begin with yourself. Individual change involves exploring how your views and values affect your thoughts, feelings, and behavior. It is not about what others think.

At the end of the day, it is still your choice about your lifestyle behaviors. This decision returns to the question about your values. What is more important to you than your life? What is more important than your health? If you feel that you have little purpose and meaning in life at the moment, you may not even care about your health. On the other hand, if you value your job and/or family more than your own life, you may sacrifice your health for external rewards and for others. Even if you value your life and health, many things may still make it difficult for you to change.

Many people believe that you have to face a life-or-death situation or hit rock bottom before changing an unhealthy habit. This belief provides the perfect excuse for not thinking about change. Nobody likes to think, *"I am slowly killing myself with my unhealthy behavior (e.g., smoking cigarettes)."* The short-term benefits of unhealthy habits (e.g., smoking to reduce stress) also make people sacrifice their long-term health (e.g., prevent disease). For example, Fred continued smoking cigarettes to relieve his stress.

An unhealthy habit is like being trapped in a locked room without a key – trapped because so much of our behavior runs on "auto pilot." To change your unhealthy habit, you have to take charge of de-programming your behavior and re-programming it into a healthy one. It takes time, effort and commitment to do "inner change." You may also need to learn more about the risks of your unhealthy habits and the benefits of change. If so, go to the library or use the World Wide Web (see Appendix B). Learning more about your behavior can help you increase your interest in changing it. Then use the exercises in this book to help you cut a key to open the door and escape! You will no longer be a prisoner of the life experiences that shaped your unhealthy behavior in the first place. For example, Susan was a single parent who felt trapped by her two small children. Let's take a look at how she used this book over several years to address some of her unhealthy habits caused by the stress of her situation.

Susan continued smoking cigarettes because it was too painful to think about quitting. She sacrificed her health to relieve the stress of being a single mother with two small children. Using this guidebook helped her better understand why she felt so trapped by nicotine addiction, but understanding her habit was only the first step. To protect her children from passive smoking, she stopped smoking in her house and avoided smoking in front of her children. She thought more seriously about quitting. Two years later, when her youngest child went off to school, she made several attempts to quit with the help of this book and the nicotine patch. She quit smoking for good a year later. When she gained eight pounds, she decided to use the book again to encourage her to exercise more and lose weight. Over the following year, she got back into better shape. She was not able to lose weight, but felt better about her body.

When Mary (her eldest daughter) was eight, she was taught about the dangers of smoking in school. She tried to persuade her grandmother to quit smoking. Susan was surprised that her mother was responsive to Mary and that she was willing to think about quitting. Susan gave the guidebook to her mother and helped her to work through it. After a year, Susan's mother quit smoking for the benefit of her grandchildren. She told them that she quit because she never wanted them to try a single cigarette.

This book can help you feel good about whatever progress you make over time, even if it is only to think more deeply about change. It can help you (and your family/friends) to work on unhealthy habits before any problems occur. But even if that happens, it's never too late to change. Even if you say or think one thing (I should quit smoking), but feel and behave differently (I enjoy smoking), this book will teach you how to do "inner" change. It can help you:

- better understand why you like to stay the same
- understand why you are having difficulties changing
- think more about change
- decide when you are ready to change
- avoid relapses back to your unhealthy habits
- act as a coach to others in helping them change

HELPING FAMILY AND FRIENDS

Whatever your success at working on inner change, you are in a better position to help others become their own health coach. However, if you simply tell family and friends to change, it can make the situation worse and lead to arguments, difficult relationships, and frustration. To avoid these situations, this book describes how you can become a motivational coach to others by working with rather than against them. By doing this, they may appreciate your help and realize how much you care about them.

When giving this book to friends or family, pick/modify any of the following suggestions, or make one up of your own. Some tips are provided to help explain the benefits of using these suggestions.

"This book has some ideas that helped me improve my health. I am concerned about your health. You may find this book helpful." (Tip – this suggestion is helpful when people appreciate your concern. But some people may interpret your well-meaning concerns as interfering in their lives. Alternatively, you could plant the seed of an idea more simply.)
"This book helped me improve my health. You might find it interesting."

"This book will help me understand why you want to continue smoking, drinking alcohol, taking drugs, not taking medications, etc." (Tip for someone not thinking about change – this suggestion will help you understand his or her thoughts, feelings, views and values better.)
 "This book will help you decide whether you want to change or not." (Tip for someone thinking about change – this suggestion may help you better understand his or her struggle to change.)

"This book will help us stop arguing about change." (Tip – this suggestion may help you avoid wasting time in arguments that are going nowhere.)

"This book will help you develop ways to prevent relapses … and help you decide whether you would like some support from me to prevent relapses." (Tip for someone who has just changed – this suggestion may help you know how to better support him or her to avoid a relapse.)

If you give someone this book as a way to tell them that they **ought to** change, they may not even look at it. Let **them** decide whether and when to work through it, with or without your help. Even if they do not change, this book can reduce your frustrations with trying to help them change.

Mrs. O. used this guidebook to become more physically active, but she was not able to persuade her overweight husband (a doctor) to do the same. After reading Chapter 6, she filled in a decision balance for her husband, but from her perspective.

Husband's reasons not to exercise	Husband's reasons to exercise
Benefits of staying the same	*Concerns about staying the same*
Prefers to watch TV rather than exercise	*Weight gain would increase his blood pressure*
Enjoys eating large meals to relax, and believes that exercise would interfere with that relaxation	*Increase risk of heart disease*
Concerns about change	*Benefits about changing*
Believes his arthritic knee pains might get worse	*Weight loss would help to lower his blood pressure and cholesterol*
Would need to find a suitable and convenient form of exercise	*Would reduce his risk of heart disease*
Resistance = 0	*Motivation = 10*

This exercise helped Mrs. O. understand how she had become more invested in helping her husband change than he had. She got so frustrated in nagging him to change that she gave up all hope of helping him lose weight and exercise more. She stopped addressing these health issues altogether.
Mrs. O. then asked her husband to fill in a decision balance for himself so that she could better understand why he did not want to exercise.

Dr. O.'s reasons not to exercise	Dr. O.'s reasons to exercise
Benefits of staying the same	Concerns about staying the same
Does not like exercise clubs	Slowly gaining weight
Does not like exercising without a purpose	My wife is concerned about my health
Concerns about change	Benefits about changing
Difficulty finding a good time to do exercise	Get into shape
Damage my knees	Lose weight and fit old clothes
Resistance = 9	Motivation = 2

Once he had completed the exercise, Dr. O. first scored his resistance and motivation based on how he felt about change. He then gave a resistance score of 6 and a motivation score of 7, based on what he thought about change. Consequently, he came to understand more clearly that he felt and thought differently about change. He also learned how his wife viewed his weight problem differently from him. This process of sharing their differences in perceptions helped Mrs. O. realize how her husband struggled with his weight and exercise issues, even though he did not appear to be concerned about them. A few months later, they decided to take up dancing lessons twice a week.

Commentary: The use of the decision balance in this manner can help families break the unproductive, circular dynamic of nagging a person to change when that person does not want to change. They can then compare and contrast the items on their decision balances and their perceptions about the change process. This process can help them to better understand their different viewpoints and work in a more cooperative, or at least a less antagonistic, manner with one another.

HELPING PROFESSIONALS

Teachers, guidance counselors, health care professionals and employers can use this guidebook on themselves before introducing it into their practice settings, wellness programs, and behavior change programs. This process will help them rapidly familiarize themselves with change concepts (e.g., resistance and motivation) and tools (e.g., the decision balance).

Having used the book on themselves, professionals can then practice using it by working with one person or a family member. In this way, they can gain first-hand experience in how people can use the tools in this book to struggle with the issue of change over time. They can thus become a health coach to themselves and a motivational coach to others. A Canadian family doctor described the benefits of using this guidebook on herself and then using this approach on one of her patients.

The examples and worksheets in the guidebook were good in terms of showing me how to do a decision balance on my need to get more exercise. Over several months, I gradually worked a daily walking program into my routine. My husband and our dog also gained benefits by joining me. It has been over 3 months and we haven't missed a day, even in bad weather.

Once I had familiarized myself with a decision balance, I also used this approach with a female patient who I have been working with for over 2 years on the dilemma of leaving her abusive husband. I asked her to fill in a decision balance and to add up the scores for staying (resistance) versus leaving the marriage (motivation). I also used these scores to help her see how she had changed her views about her marital relationship over time. The decision balance helped her to put her reasons for staying versus her reasons for leaving her husband in a concrete form; she saw more clearly that she was ready to make this big step She was finally able to get her own apartment and move out. She surprised herself with how strong she was. She also had good support from her adult son, her employer and several friends.

This example highlights the benefits of addressing both personal and professional issues in learning how to help people change. Counselors and health care professionals can learn more sophisticated ways of using this approach by reading the books *Beyond Advice: 1. Becoming a Motivational Practitioner, and 2. Developing Motivational Skills.* In addition, Web-based training and small group workshops can help counselors and health care professionals become more skillful in developing more individualized approaches for people. Even then, counselors and health care professionals may need to seek out specialists to help people change, particularly when people have mental health problems, severe addictions, or difficult relationship problems.

GETTING PROFESSIONAL HELP

Professional help may be needed if you, your family or friend cannot change using this self-help or mutual help approach. A health professional trained in motivational approaches to behavior change may help you, but you may need a specialist's help if you have mental health problems, or alcohol and drug addiction.

Filling in the decision balance below may help you decide if you need professional help. It is a relatively easy task to write out what you think are your answers to the questions listed in the decision balance below. However, it may not capture how you feel about getting professional help. Negative emotions, such as fear, anger and anxiety, may stop you from getting the help that you need to be healthy. But, by avoiding professional help, you do not have to deal with these negative emotions. It takes courage to recognize and deal with these emotions that prevent you from getting professional help to feel better. For this reason, it may be important for you to ask yourself this question as well: How do you feel about getting professional help?

Deciding Whether to Get Professional Help

Reasons for using self-help/mutual help approach	Reasons for seeking professional help
What are the advantages of using a self-help/mutual help approach?	*What are the disadvantages about relying on a self-help/mutual help approach?*
What are the disadvantages about seeking professional help?	*What are the advantages of getting professional help?*

HOW TO USE THIS GUIDEBOOK

Section A prepares you to address your unhealthy habits. Chapter 1 helps you assess your readiness to change your unhealthy habits. If you know what habit you want to change, skip to Chapter 2. If you are really eager to change (for example, to quit smoking), go straight to Section B (Chapters 3-5).

Section B helps you to become your own health coach. This section is divided into three chapters:
      3. Get Ready for Change
      4. Take Charge of Your Health
      5. Make Plans for Change

If you are eager and ready to change, read Chapters 3-4 quickly and spend more time on Chapter 5. For example, if you are a smoker and are ready to quit, Chapter 5 can help you learn about treating nicotine addiction and preventing relapses. These chapters provide many learning exercises to help you change. You may find some exercises more helpful than others. As you become familiar with the different options, you will learn which ones work best for you. You can also use your progress and goal charts to monitor change over time.

Section C can help you become a coach to family and friends. Chapter 6 describes how to become a motivational coach to family and friends with unhealthy habits. You can share what you have learned to help them work through this book. Then, invite them to assess their health behaviors and read the book. On the other hand, if you want additional support to change your own behavior, consider asking someone else to read Chapter 6. Chapter 7 describes how to become a preventive coach for your children. You can help them develop healthy habits and avoid starting unhealthy ones.

Although you can read this book in one sitting, it is better to do a few exercises at a time. Do the exercises at a pace that works for you. You decide which ones to do and when. Many exercises are worth doing more than once. You can pick sections of the book to re-read, to address particular issues that are important to you.

Any past failures at changing an unhealthy habit may make you feel discouraged and hopeless. These feelings can make you feel like giving up altogether. But you will succeed if you **never quit trying to quit.** With each "failure," you learn something new about your unhealthy habit that you can use when you try again. People vary widely in how quickly they change. Some can take a giant leap forward in a few days and others take years to change.

Write directly in this guidebook, or keep a separate journal or diary. A journal can keep your notes private and make it easier to look back over them. Whether or not you write directly in this book, consider making a copy of the decision balance (see p. 40). Your decision balance is the most important tool to help you think about change.

In brief, decide for yourself how you can best use this book. You can work with any of the following options: alone, or with support from family members and/or friends, the Web and the Internet, and lay health organizations and helping professionals. The latter two groups may wish to organize small groups or voluntary coaches, or provide telephone support counseling. And remember, not everyone can change without professional help. This book also helps you decide whether or not to seek professional help.

SECTION A:
UNHEALTHY HABITS

We live in a disease-producing society. Worldwide, smoking is on the increase, and alcohol problems are not going away. We have not won the war on drugs. Lack of exercise and being overweight also are major health problems. Children who watch more television exercise less and weigh more. Such unhealthy habits are a major source of illness, as a former U.S. Surgeon General noted:

> *Diseases are of two types: Those we develop inadvertently, and those we bring on ourselves by failure to practice preventive measures. Preventable illness makes [up] approximately 70% of the burden of illness and associated costs.*
>
> C. Everett Koop, 1995

This section of the guidebook first explores why people keep their unhealthy habits and then addresses what affects whether or not people can and will change such behavior.

WHY DO PEOPLE KEEP THEIR UNHEALTHY HABITS?

People do so because they:
- May not fully know the risks of their behavior
  "I didn't know that smoking caused heart disease."
- Wish to minimize future risks and harm
  "It won't happen to me."
- Ignore the health risks
  "I know it causes harm, but I am not going to think about it."
- Feel hopeless about changing their behavior
  "I feel hopeless about quitting because . . ."
- Feel it's out of their control to change
  "Nicotine addiction controls me."
- Deny their health risks and believe that God will take care of them
  "My health is in God's hands, and He will look after me."
- Believe that their fate is already determined
  "My days are numbered, and there is nothing I can do about it."
- Think that the "good times" are more important than "good health"
  "I only live once, so let the good times roll."
- Take pleasure in or even boast about their habits
  "Coffee and cigars are the best way to finish a good meal."

PROMOTE HEALTH, NOT DISEASE

Unhealthy habits (such as not eating well, not exercising enough, being overweight, smoking, drinking too much alcohol, or using illegal drugs) will claim more lives in the future than all the wars in the past. Former Secretary of Health Joseph Califano says that you can make a huge difference:

We are killing ourselves by our own careless habits. You, the individual, can do more for your own health and well-being than any doctor, any hospital, any drug, or any exotic medical device.

We may minimize, ignore, or deny that we live in a disease-producing society. Regrettably, this is because we do not know what it is like to live in a health-promoting society. For example, tobacco companies are far more effective in producing diseases than health care systems are in preventing them.

Two questions can help us think about this further. How does a fish discover that it lives in water? If the water were polluted, how could a fish know whether the water was unhealthy? The answer to both questions is that a fish does not know it lives in water, let alone in a polluted environment. But we, as individual humans, can learn that the water is polluted (disease-producing), and that we need to purify it (promote health). Governments, ethical companies, schools, workplaces, and health care settings can help us change from a disease-producing to a health-promoting society. Divided, we fail and produce disease. United, we could promote health for all.

However, you cannot wait until these groups develop ideal programs. This workbook will help you and others to understand and change your unhealthy habits, or at least understand each other better if either of you find change difficult. For example, you may not lose the amount of weight that you want to lose, but if you exercise regularly, reduce your stress level, increase your sense of well-being, and come to terms with your body size, you can still improve your health and feel better about who you are.

In Chapter 1, you will learn to distinguish between "good times," which do not promote healthy habits, and the "good life," which does. You will also find out how to develop the kinds of healthy habits that lead to a good life. Chapter 2 explores the many factors involved in hindering and helping to motivate you to change and enables you to decide whether or not you are ready to change.

CHAPTER 1:
WHAT ARE THE GOOD TIMES AND GOOD LIFE TO YOU?

To help you answer this question, the table below lists some differences between "good-time" and "good-life" people.

Good-time People	Good-life People
Want instant gratification	Invest in long-term well-being
Think that the short-term benefits are worth more than long-term benefits	Think that the long-term benefits are worth more than short-term benefits
Avoid struggles with learning and growing	Strive to learn and to grow
Avoid stresses and difficult situations	Address stresses and difficult situations
Let go of their responsibilities carelessly	Let go of their responsibilities carefully

WHO SELLS YOU THE GOOD TIMES?

What do you need for the good times? Can you enjoy life without relying on so many things, particularly the unhealthy ones? Who decides what is healthy and unhealthy for you? Do you simply accept what others suggest are the good times? How do you decide what is good for you? In answering these questions, the media, advertisements, multinational companies, family and friends all shape what you think are the good times.

They teach you that the world of things is more important than the world of being. What you have (possessions and money) is more important than who you are. The economy focuses much more on the production and consumption of things (e.g., cigarettes, cigars, and alcohol needed for relaxation and the good times) than on new ways of being. Modern science and research funding also focuses more on things (curing diseases) and outer-space exploration (dating the beginning of the cosmos) than on being (enhancing self-understanding) and behavioral change (promoting health).

We have become so caught up in studying, producing, or doing things that we have lost touch with our being. Our outer lives have become more important than our inner lives. We seek what others tell us is necessary for the good life: tobacco products, alcohol, drugs, and products that enhance our beauty, appearance, and prestige. Self-image becomes the idol.

In addition, many people need to escape from bad feelings (anger, depression, or low self-esteem) and bad situations (family difficulties, unemployment, or work stress).

They use quick fixes (drugs, alcohol or overeating) for short-term comfort and for coping with these situations.

Unhealthy habits may thus result from giving higher priorities to short-term rather than to long-term benefits, from not investing in one's future, and from neglecting oneself. These habits are a measure of how much more we value the idols of image, instant pleasure, and convenience, as opposed to our health. The question is, can we create a health-promoting society? In addition to studying, producing, and consuming things, we need to understand ourselves better and develop a more balanced approach to health and the good life. In other words, we cannot assess the strengths of a society only by its achievements; we also need to look at how the overall population takes care of itself and behaves in healthy ways, despite its problems.

WHAT IS THE GOOD LIFE?

When people live only in the present and feel that they have no future, then their "good life" is really only "good times" or what they feel now. This lifestyle can be full of many shortsighted, unhealthy pleasures. These behaviors damage long-term health and shorten the time available to enjoy a really good life. Good-life people, on the other hand, take simple pleasure in life, are passionate about life pursuits, and thrive on developing relationships, self-sufficiency, and new abilities. A caring community and family can help you develop a good life, but it is ultimately up to you.

A good life is when you take care of your mind, body, and soul. A healthy soul helps you to clarify your values, meaning, and purpose in life, and deepens your connections to others, the community, higher powers, faith, or beliefs. Your soul is your guiding light to a healthy mind and body. Likewise, a healthy mind helps you to manage stress and negative emotions (depression, anxiety, low self-esteem, and anger) and to take care of your body by:

- Not smoking, drinking alcohol excessively, or using illegal drugs
- Eating a balanced diet, keeping your weight under control, and exercising regularly
- Wearing protective gear (safety belts, bicycle and motorbike helmets, protective eyeglasses for some work and sports activities)
- Practicing safe sex to avoid sexually transmitted diseases
- Using contraception to avoid unwanted pregnancy
- Taking drugs as prescribed by your doctor

We cannot be good-life people all the time, but we can work toward this goal.

WHY ARE HEALTHY HABITS IMPORTANT FOR THE GOOD LIFE?

To increase your chance of becoming a "good-life" person, you need to develop healthy habits and change unhealthy ones.

A. Develop Healthy Habits

The following section lists some areas where you can make changes to improve your health. You can also add your own areas of change.

1. Exercise regularly

Any form of physical activity (walking, running, biking, dancing, sports) for about 20 minutes per day can make you feel good, improve your quality of sleep, and increase your energy. Exercise that makes you sweat can give you a natural "high." Exercise can protect you not only against depression, anxiety, and the effects of stress, but also improve your physical health.

Regular exercise can lower blood pressure. It prevents weight gain, heart disease, cancer of the large bowel (colon), bone thinning (osteoporosis), non-insulin dependent diabetes, and hip fractures, as well as helping people with osteoarthritis function better. Diabetic patients can lower their glucose levels if they exercise regularly.

In spite of these health benefits, some people say that they do not have the time or are too tired to exercise. But getting into shape can actually increase your energy! If you do not like to exercise, try to find another activity that is fun for you: dancing, gardening, hiking in the country, walking and talking with a friend, or any sport.

2. Eat a balanced diet

Eating unhealthy food and too much food can cause major health problems and increase your risk of dying from heart disease and some cancers, such as colon and breast cancer. Modern diets are energy-dense: high fat, high sugars (such as glucose), low fiber, and low complex carbohydrates, i.e., starch. Many fast food restaurants serve such diets.

A healthy diet can reverse the risk of developing some diseases. Such a diet consists of high fiber, high complex carbohydrates, high antioxidants (such as vitamin E), high folic acid, frequent intake of fruits, vegetables, cereals, and legumes, low fat (particularly animal fats), and low sugar.

In addition, there are low-fat, low-cholesterol, low-salt, American Heart Association, or American Diabetic Association diets. Read a book on nutrition and dieting, or talk to a dietitian, nutritionist or health care professional about any special diet. Call the American Dietetic Association Hotline (1-800-366-1555), or refer to the Web sites in Appendix B for further information.

3. Keep your weight under control

Different cultural practices also affect the weight of a given population. A brief example will help to explain this relationship better. Many Western European visitors to the United States immediately notice the large food portions in restaurants. As a general rule, this is because in America value for money is measured more by meal size than by health benefits. Not surprisingly, visitors also notice that the percentage of overweight people is much higher in the United States than in their own countries. In fact, from the 1960s to the 1990s, the percentage of overweight, middle-aged Americans rose from 17% to 32%.

The following story further highlights differences in cultural practices. An overweight Irish cook flew on the cheapest flight (off-season) to New York City once a year. She went on a shopping spree for oversized clothes, enough to last her the year. It was much cheaper to do this than to buy expensive oversized clothes in Ireland where the percentage of overweight people is much smaller. This short story illustrates how some cultures promote overeating and cater to overweight people, while others do not. However, culture is not the only factor that influences the weight of individuals. Your food intake, level of physical activity, and family history of obesity (genetic make-up) all affect your weight.

Being overweight can have a number of long-term health consequences: high blood pressure, heart disease, non-insulin dependent diabetes, and arthritis. It is better to try to prevent weight gain in the first place since it is more difficult to lose weight after you have gained it. Long-term success in maintaining weight loss is also difficult. Many people lose weight in the short term, but only about 10% can maintain long-term weight loss. Even if you stay the same weight, you can be fit and get into shape.

4. Use seat belts in cars and crash helmets on motorbikes

Laws mandating the use of seat belts in cars and crash helmets while on motorbikes have significantly reduced death rates and severe injuries in accidents.

5. Use prescription drugs as prescribed

Up to 50% of people do not consistently take their prescription drugs for treating chronic diseases such as high blood pressure and high cholesterol. They need to take them regularly.

6. Practice safe sex to prevent disease

Safe sex practices (using condoms) can prevent sexually transmitted diseases and AIDS. This issue is very important when young people become sexually active. There are only three ways to be safe. 1. Don't have sex. 2. Use a condom every time. 3. Stay in one relationship with a partner who is free of sexually transmitted diseases.

7. Use contraception to prevent pregnancy

Unplanned pregnancy is a significant problem, particularly among teenagers. Abstinence or contraception can prevent young people from having unwanted children.

B. Change Unhealthy Habits

This section lists some of the unhealthy habits that threaten your health or those of your family and friends. You can add other behaviors to the list, such as poor dental care (e.g., not flossing teeth), gambling, lack of skin protection against sun exposure, failure to have eye and hearing tests, and lack of self-care of chronic diseases.

1. Stop tobacco use

Tobacco is addictive because it contains nicotine. Smoking is the most serious and damaging habit for you and others. It can cause cancer, heart conditions, lung disease, peptic ulcer, and low birth weight if women smoke during pregnancy. There is only one recommendation: stop all tobacco use.

Second-hand smoke also increases health risks for other family members, such as increasing the risk for bronchitis, middle ear infections, and even sudden infant death syndrome. If smokers cannot quit but wish to protect nonsmoking family members, they can smoke outside the house and other enclosed areas.

2. Don't drink alcohol excessively

The amount of alcohol that people drink may vary over time. Types of drinking may fit into any of the following groups: abstinence, low-risk use, hazardous use, harmful use (abuse) of alcohol, and dependent use. The percentage of the population with alcohol abuse and dependence is about 15%-20% and 5%, respectively.

It is difficult to be certain what level of alcohol use is safe for adults. However, the U.S. National Institute of Alcohol Abuse and Alcoholism (NIAAA) made the following recommendations. Men are at risk for health problems if they have more than 14 drinks in a week or more than four drinks on one occasion. Nonpregnant women are at risk for health problems if they have more than seven drinks (12 grams of alcohol) per week or more than three drinks on any one occasion. Pregnant women are advised not to drink alcohol.

Other countries vary in how they define low-risk drinking because of controversy about how to set a limit. Appendix C lists the recommendations for low-risk drinking in three countries.

Hazardous use of alcohol is defined as drinking more than low-risk limits but without evidence of harm or dependency. People who drink at this level are at increased risk for developing alcohol abuse and dependency, particularly if they increase their consumption over time.

Harmful use of alcohol is defined as drinking that causes any negative medical, psychological, or social problems. Use a self-assessment measure to help you decide whether you, a family member, or a friend has an alcohol abuse and/or dependency problem (see Appendix D). Some people can stop drinking alcohol by themselves, but others need professional help and/or the support of Alcoholics Anonymous.

Drinking too much alcohol increases your risk of developing stomach problems, high blood pressure, liver disease, pancreatitis, missing work days, minor injuries at home and work, road traffic accidents, and relationship problems. It also increases your risk of dying from cancers (liver, stomach, and breast), stroke (hemorrhage), and suicide.

3. Don't use illegal drugs
Illegal drug use is often associated with excessive alcohol use and smoking. Drugs such as cocaine, amphetamines, and methamphetamine are stimulants. People use them for many different reasons: excitement or escaping from, or coping with, life problems. None of these drugs improve people's health, but most users feel their short-term benefits are worth the risks.

4. Be environmentally responsible
Environmental issues (such as pollution, poor sanitation, waste products, and energy conservation) will become the most important health issue in the world over the next one hundred years. It will take both individual and collective responsibility to arrest and reverse environmental damage and the health hazards that result.

ANY CONCERNS ABOUT YOUR HEALTH BEHAVIORS?

The checklist below will help you assess your health behaviors and your readiness to change them.

Circle a response to each health decision using the letter code N or Y.
N = not applicable to me.
Y = yes. For each yes response, circle the "readiness-to-change" scale:
1 = not thinking about change
2 = thinking about change
3 = preparing to change

Health Behavior Checklist

Self-assessment of health behaviors	Response		Readiness to change		
1. I do not exercise enough	N	Y	1	2	3
2. I have unhealthy eating habits	N	Y	1	2	3
3. I am overweight	N	Y	1	2	3
4. I do not put on my seat belt in my car every time	N	Y	1	2	3
5. I sometimes forget to take prescription drugs	N	Y	1	2	3
6. I do not practice safe sex every time	N	Y	1	2	3
7. I sometimes forget to use contraception	N	Y	1	2	3
8. I use tobacco products	N	Y	1	2	3

9. I drink alcohol more than
    For men: 14 drinks per week
    For women: 7 drinks per week
	N N	Y Y	1 1	2 2	3 3

10. I use illegal drugs	N	Y	1	2	3
11. I can do more to protect the environment	N	Y	1	2	3
12. Add your own example*	N	Y	1	2	3
How many health behaviors do you want to address?					

*For example: I work too hard; I do not have enough "play time" to enjoy life (trapped by work demands); I need to learn how to do nothing without driving myself crazy; I overeat, gain weight, and do not exercise on business trips away from home; I lack sleep; I am too stressed; I don't make time for hobbies, relaxation, or yoga regularly; I bite my nails.

Once you have completed the checklist, you are ready to prioritize and move toward change.

DECIDING WHETHER TO THINK ABOUT CHANGE

Many factors can affect whether you are willing to think about change. For example, if you have more than one unhealthy habit, you may:

- Feel differently about whether and when you are ready to change each behavior.
- Feel more hopeful about changing one behavior compared to another.

The following questions can help you decide which unhealthy habit to address first:

- Which behavior is most important to change in order to improve your health? Which is the next most important one to change?
- Which is the easiest behavior to change? Which is the next one?
- Is there a difference in your priorities between the most important and the easiest behavior to change?

You will learn more about yourself if you work on one behavior at a time. Sometimes, it helps to learn by addressing an easier behavior to change (stop nail biting) before addressing a more difficult one (quit drinking). This may help you overcome your fear of addressing more challenging health issues. Whatever you do, you are more likely to succeed if you continue to think about change. Build on your successes and use them to address other behaviors.

If you feel hopeless and powerless to change, you will probably not change. But these feelings can provide opportunities to learn and understand something really important about yourself. Even if you think that you will fail, try to make a small change so you can understand your feelings better. You can set yourself up to fail by setting unrealistic goals (e.g., lose 50 pounds in six months). Think about a reasonable goal. Some success will come if you keep trying to reach some goal. Each "failure" provides another opportunity to learn what it would take for you to change. Whatever you learn about changing yourself is an achievement!

CHAPTER 2:
UNDERSTANDING CHANGE

If you learn about how to change before trying to change your behavior, you will be more successful in the long run. Chapter 2 will help you:
- Understand how unhealthy and healthy forces affect whether you change.
- Understand how you view change.
- Prepare you to become your own health coach.

UNHEALTHY AND HEALTHY FORCES FOR CHANGE

Internal and external factors can affect whether you change. The internal factors are your resistance and motivation to change. Resistance is all your reasons for behaving in unhealthy ways. Motivation is all your reasons for behaving in healthy ways. External factors are the barriers and supports that relate to work, family, school, and social situations. Barriers can promote unhealthy behaviors or create difficulties in developing healthy ones. Supports (people, materials, or community resources) promote healthy behaviors and prevent unhealthy ones.

A simple framework can help you understand healthy and unhealthy forces for change (see Figure 2.1). You will develop healthy habits if your motivation and supports, which are your healthy forces for change, are greater than your resistance and barriers, which are your unhealthy forces for change. The reverse is also true.

Figure 2.1: Force for Change Model

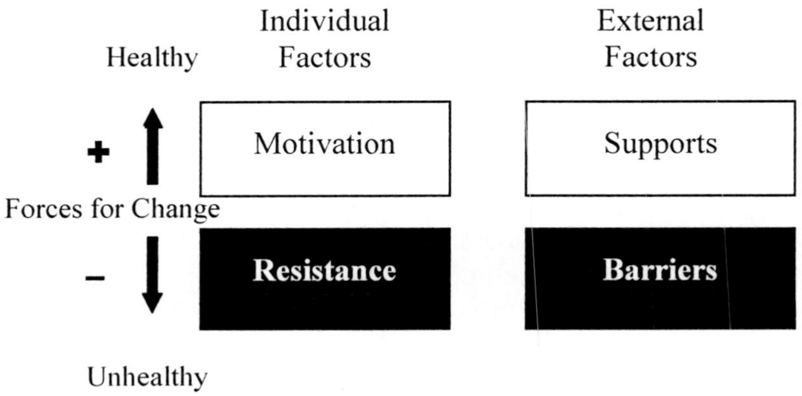

The following example illustrates how different internal and external factors can affect the force for change.

Mrs. P. and her 17-year-old daughter, Kathy, are both smokers who live together in an apartment. Mrs. P. wants her daughter to quit smoking with her, but her daughter does not want to. The table below lists the internal and external factors that affect change for Mrs. P.

Factors Affecting the Forces for Change

Force for Change	Internal Factors	External Factors
Healthy Force	Motivation Stop getting chronic bronchitis. Not get shortness of breath when walking. Save money (particularly if cigarette tax goes up).	Supports Kathy supports her mother's attempts to quit. Grandparents want Kathy and Mrs. P. to quit.
Unhealthy Force	Resistance Help her to cope with stress. Lack willpower to quit because of nicotine addiction. Withdrawal symptoms make her stress worse.	Barriers Kathy will still be smoking at home. Stressful life and family situations.

The relative strengths of these two forces influence whether Mrs. P. will think more about quitting, or even quit.

A. External Factors

To help achieve your goals, you need to increase your supports and overcome the barriers to change, if possible. However, some people use their barriers or the lack of support as excuses not to change: "My boss is stressing me out, so why should I quit smoking? It helps me cope." The following brief discussions about barriers and supports may help you to understand why people develop, avoid changing, or change their unhealthy habits.

Increase your supports for change

Support can help promote healthy habits or encourage changing unhealthy ones. But does support always help adults change their behavior? For example, family support has different influences on men and women who have diabetes. It has been shown that women who are satisfied with their social support achieve better control of their diabetes than women who are less satisfied. In contrast, men who are satisfied with their social support have less control of their diabetes than men who are less satisfied with their

24

social support. These findings raise issues about how men and women need different kinds of support to deal with a chronic disease. Well-meaning family members can make the situation worse. Thus, you may have to clarify what kinds of support are helpful or unhelpful for yourself and others before you decide to change.

Overcome barriers to change

Barriers can make it more difficult for you to change your unhealthy habits or even prevent you from changing. These barriers include overwork (housework and/or employment), money problems, family stresses, work stress, negative peer pressure, transportation problems, and unsafe school or housing situations. Recognizing, reducing, and overcoming these barriers can help you achieve your goals for change.

Family, work, religion, and school are all external factors that can create supports and barriers to develop or change your unhealthy habit. For example, teenagers whose parents and peers smoke (barrier) are much more likely to smoke than teenagers who have nonsmoking parents and friends (support). Smoking parents and peers provide ready access to cigarettes and act as role models in encouraging teenagers to develop a smoking habit.

As adults, smokers are more likely to marry smokers. Smokers who are married to a nonsmoker or an ex-smoker are more likely to quit and remain abstinent. But nagging families and friends can be barriers as it makes it less likely that a smoker will quit. In fact, you will increase your chance of changing if you thank your family for their concern and politely tell them that nagging will not work.

You also can help family and friends avoid becoming frustrated with you by explaining to them that you are not ready for change. Again, thank them for their concern and let them know whether, when, and WHAT KIND of support you may need.

B. Internal Factors

Even if you cannot change your supports and barriers, you can learn how to change your behavior. Following are three ways of understanding how motivation and resistance (internal factors) influence whether or not you change your unhealthy habits. Chapter 4 describes in more detail how to reduce your resistance and increase your motivation to change, independent of any external factors.

1. Understanding Your Readiness to Change

Motivation (see decision balance on next page) is your reasons to change: the pros of change. It involves your concerns about the consequences of an unhealthy behavior (for example, developing chronic bronchitis caused by smoking) and the benefits of adopting a healthy behavior (for example, walking without feeling short of breath).

Resistance is your reasons to stay the same: the cons of change. It involves your concerns about the consequences of adopting a healthy behavior (nicotine withdrawal symptoms make stress worse) and the benefits from the unhealthy behavior (cigarettes help to relieve stress).

Decision Balance

Choice A: Reasons to stay the same	*Choice B: Reasons to change*
Benefits of staying the same	*Concerns about staying the same*
Concerns about change	*Benefits of change*
Resistance *(Cons of change)*	*Motivation* *(Pros of change)*

The pros and cons affect whether you are ready to change. Readiness to change is divided into five stages. Your views about the pros and cons change as you work through these stages.

Stage 1 – Not considering change

You may not think about change for many different reasons. At one extreme, you may not know that your behavior is harmful to your health. At the other extreme, you may know all about these harms but decide not to change. A diehard smoker is an example of such a person. You may also not think about change for a variety of other reasons: too stressed, feeling depressed, or having too much to do.

As long as you view your reasons to stay the same (left column of decision balance) as being more important than your reasons to change (right column of decision balance), the cons outweigh the pros. You have no reason to think about change. In contrast, family members and friends often view your situation the other way around; they view the pros as outweighing the cons. They treat you as though you ought to change, even if you are not thinking about it.

Stage 2 – Considering change

If you view your reasons to change and to stay the same as equally important, the pros and cons of change are in balance. You will think about behavior change. You feel as if you are stuck or going in circles. You have mixed feelings about change. You often change your mind about what to do. These feelings and thoughts are signs of progress. Do not get discouraged. For example, smokers may think about quitting for 1-2 years before they finally quit. The learning exercises in this workbook can help you change more quickly.

Stage 3 – Preparing to change

When you view your reasons to change as more important than your reasons to stay the same, the pros outweigh the cons. No longer feeling stuck, you can push ahead to set a date to change, starting in a month or so.

Stage 4 – Changing your unhealthy behavior

Your goal for change may range from short-term, small changes, to long-term, ideal goals. You need to set a reasonable goal for change that you feel is within your reach. For example, select a short-term (2-4 weeks) goal of low-risk drinking or abstinence. You can then use the experience of working on this short-term goal to help you decide about your long-term goals.

Stage 5 – Keep doing it

You can use different means to prevent lapses and relapses. A lapse is a temporary setback, such as smoking a couple of cigarettes over a few days. A relapse occurs when you return to your old habit, such as smoking a pack of cigarettes daily. Many factors can trigger a lapse or relapse: negative or positive feelings, tempting situations, and stressful events (divorce, unemployment, work pressure, and family difficulties). You are in the maintenance stage if you are able to keep to your goal for six months or more.

Recycle

You may not move through these stages (listed above) in sequence. You may recycle through them several times before achieving your long-term goal. For example, smokers who quit without professional help have usually made at least three serious attempts before they quit for good. You can use these stages to monitor your progress over time.

2. Understanding Your Motives to Change

Your list of reasons to change may not really explain your motives to change. Are those reasons really yours? You are more likely to change if you have freely chosen the reasons rather than simply accepting what others have told you. Place your reasons to change in the four groups described below. You can also track whether you change your motives over time.

Indifference

"I don't care to do it," "I've got better things to do," or "I don't care if I live or die" are examples of indifference. You may not want change because of a variety of factors: stress; depression; difficult family, home, or work situations; financial problems; relationship problems; or death of family or friends. You may need to come to terms with these factors before trying to change.

Controlling external reasons

You change mainly because of family, friends, or health care professionals. For example, "I am changing because my family wants me to." A genuine sense of free choice may be absent in your decision. You may feel pressured to change and do not want to upset others. You are unlikely to maintain your long-term goals, particularly if others stop encouraging you to change.

Controlling internal reasons

Although it may appear as though you are changing for freely chosen reasons, you act more out of a sense of obligation. You say to yourself: "I **should, must, or ought** to change." You are not fully committed to change. You may even feel conflicted, anxious, or guilty about not changing. If you change only because of these reasons, you are less likely to achieve your goals over the long term. Any change is dependent on you continuing to say to yourself: "I should, must, or ought to stick to this goal."

Freely chosen reasons

You feel a true sense of free choice about whether to change. For example, "I love to exercise because it makes me feel great and I have more energy," or "I'm going to stick to my goal because it is really important to me." You change because of your views and values, not because of someone else's views and values. You change without a sense of duty, obligation, or a need for control coming from yourself or others. Although support from others can help, your personal choice is the driving force for change.

3. Understanding Your Confidence and Ability to Change

Your confidence and ability can affect whether you try to change your habits. For example, if you lack confidence about your ability to change or fear that you may fail, you may not even try to change. On the other hand, failure can help you learn what it would take to develop your confidence and ability. Failure is an opportunity to learn about change, not to put yourself down.

Your confidence and ability are different from your belief about whether you can reach your goal for change. For example, Mr. D. had the ability and felt confident about keeping to a low-calorie diet and an exercise program. However, he did not think that he would lose 30 pounds over two years. Consequently, Mr. D. did not bother changing because he thought that he could not reach this goal. An overly ambitious goal can be used as an excuse for not trying to change.

ASSESS YOUR CHANCES OF CHANGING

Now that you understand some of the factors that affect whether or not you can change, it is time to see what your chances of making a successful change are. Below is a checklist that can help you think about this issue. Pick one behavior, such as smoking, that you want to address and assess your chances of changing, using the scale below. Your chances of long-term change increase the more you strongly agree with the following ten statements.

1 = Strongly Agree; 2 = Agree; 3 = Neutral; 4 = Disagree; 5 = Strongly Disagree.

Assess Your Chances of Changing Please circle the appropriate number based on the above scale.	
1. My unhealthy behavior is serious and of concern to me.	1 2 3 4 5
2. I believe that my behavior puts my health at risk.	1 2 3 4 5
3. I explore both the reasons to change and not to change.	1 2 3 4 5
4. Reasons to change are more important than reasons to stay the same.	1 2 3 4 5
5. I have freely chosen my reasons to change.	1 2 3 4 5
6. I have the confidence and ability to change.	1 2 3 4 5
7. I feel that I can achieve my goal for change.	1 2 3 4 5
8. I can reduce the barriers and enhance the supports to change.	1 2 3 4 5
9. I can ask others for support when I need it.	1 2 3 4 5
10. I will use support from others if provided.	1 2 3 4 5

After reading Chapter 3, you may want to reconsider your responses to these statements.

SECTION B:
BECOME YOUR OWN HEALTH COACH

After filling out the checklist assessing your chance of changing, pick an unhealthy behavior you may want to change. This guidebook will help you break this unhealthy habit and learn how to develop a healthy one. Good and bad habits often run on automatic pilot. Because we learn and develop unhealthy habits over so many years, we can lose touch with why we do what we do. It takes time, energy, and work to change these habits.

As you read though Section B, work at a pace that suits your situation. Keep an eye on your "excuses" for not working on change. Your excuses will help you understand why you do not change. This is an important step toward change.

Chapter 3 will help you to get ready for change if you are not yet sure you want to change. Chapter 4 can help you take charge of your health. Once you are ready and eager for change, Chapter 5 will help you put a plan for change into action. Together, these chapters provide a menu of learning exercises that will help you become your own health coach.

A chart at the end of each chapter helps you to keep a record of the dates when you used the exercises and your assessment of their usefulness. You may discover that some exercises will be more helpful than others at different times. For example, as you think about change, you may give higher scores to the exercises in Chapter 3 than in Chapter 5. As you begin to make a change, you may give higher scores to the exercises in Chapter 5. If you fail to make progress in changing your behavior, it may help to work through some earlier exercises again.

USE THE SEED CYCLE

As you work through the following exercises, you can sow your own "seeds" to develop healthy habits. The SEED cycle helps you make and measure progress. This cycle consists of four steps:

1. **S**tudy - select an exercise to read
2. **E**xercise - write out a response to the exercise
3. **E**valuate - assess the helpfulness of the exercise
4. **D**ocument - use the progress and goal charts (Appendix A) to monitor the impact of using the exercise over time

You can use this cycle repeatedly to make progress over time. Some people only need a few seeds, but others need to sow lots of seeds to see which ones will grow. Here are some questions to ask yourself as you complete each exercise:

1. Study – Which learning exercise did you read about?

Change can take time. You decide the pace at which to study the exercises in Chapters 3-5; you don't need to read them all at once.

2. Exercise – Which learning exercise did you write about?

Writing out responses to the learning exercises is more effective in helping you change than just reading about them. You may skip any exercise and come back to it later. A chart at the end of each chapter helps you to track which ones you used.

3. Evaluate – How helpful was this exercise?

Each learning exercise has a rating box to record your opinion about using it. After completing an exercise and writing out a response to it, pick any number between 0-10 using the scale provided (see below) to rate the helpfulness of the exercise.

0	1	2	3	4	5	6	7	8	9	10
Not helpful					Moderately helpful					Very helpful

After completing a chapter, you can transfer your scores from these boxes and record them in the chart at the end of each chapter. These charts help you monitor how helpful the exercises were. Some exercises can be more helpful if you repeat them over time. You can use the exercises again at a later date and monitor whether their helpfulness changes.

When you have difficulty changing your behavior, you can review these charts. Check which exercises you missed, or where you had a low score. You may have missed an opportunity to think about change in new ways.

4. Document – What impact did the learning exercise have on you?

Are these exercises increasing your understanding about your unhealthy habit and the opportunity for change? You can use the progress and goal charts (Appendix A) provided to document and monitor the effectiveness of using these exercises over time. Your notes can also help you identify what you are learning that is new about yourself. Looking back over your notes can also help you learn more about what it would take for you to make further progress toward your goals for change.

MONITORING CHANGE OVER TIME

Before using the exercises in Chapters 3-5, turn to the progress chart in Appendix A now (page 117). Score your resistance, motivation, competing priorities, energy, motives, confidence, and ability to change, using the 0-10 scale. As you complete the exercises, you can return to this chart and assess in what ways this guidebook helped you change any of your scores. In other words, the progress chart can help you monitor how you change over time. Your progress chart can also help you assess whether these exercises are helping you to work toward your goals of change.

CHAPTER 3:
GET READY FOR CHANGE

Now select one of your unhealthy habits. For this behavior, are you:
> A. Not considering change?
> B. Considering change?
> C. Preparing to change?

This chapter is particularly helpful if you are not yet thinking about change, as well as if you are thinking about or preparing to change. You will know more about what drives you to behave in unhealthy ways and about what may cause you to relapse after you have changed.

You can use any of the following exercises to think about change. Do as many or as few of them as you want. After writing out a response to any exercise, pick a number between 0-10 using the same scale as before to rate the helpfulness of the exercise. Put your score in the box provided below the exercise. Leave the boxes in the right-hand margin empty if you do not write a response to the question posed in any particular exercise. Select only **one** unhealthy habit at a time when doing these learning exercises.

1. LIST THE BENEFITS OF YOUR UNHEALTHY HABIT

You will be more effective in making changes if you understand the benefits of your unhealthy habit. It can be difficult to make such a list because you may have forgotten about some of the benefits of the habit, which is what stops you from changing it. Because this is so important in helping you to change, the following exercise will help you in the first step toward filling out a decision balance. Two examples will be used throughout to help you understand the importance of thinking about the different benefits of an unhealthy habit, in this case smoking.

Mrs. G. decided to quit smoking. A month later, her husband left her and wanted a divorce. She felt so angry toward her husband that she wanted to smoke again. She came to understand more fully that she smoked cigarettes whenever she got angry. She decided not to let her husband get the better of her. Instead of smoking to reduce her anger about the divorce, she expressed her anger appropriately by talking to friends and her lawyer. She thought that if she could quit now, she would cope better with any future stress. In effect, she used her anger to improve her physical and psychological health instead of acting in ways that could make it worse.

34

Mr. B. did not recognize how much he smoked to cope with feelings of sadness, frustration, and irritability caused by work stress. When he quit smoking, his wife even suggested that he move out for a while because he was so difficult to live with. In contrast, Mr. B. was not fully aware of these emotional changes until well after he quit smoking. A year after quitting, he understands more fully how difficult he was to live with, and how much he had depended on cigarettes to cope with work stress. It took him a year to learn how to cope with these feelings in ways that did not irritate his wife.

In the following exercise, a checklist of benefits can help you understand the driving force for your unhealthy habit. These benefits include lifestyle, emotional, relational, coping, work-related, social and spiritual reasons. Since some benefits may not be relevant to your unhealthy behavior – for example, lack of exercise may not have any work-related benefits – check off the relevant ones only. Comparing how Mrs. G. and Mr. B. used these checklists may make it easier to complete yours.

Mrs. G. was very attuned to her benefits from smoking. On a quick review of the checklists, she easily identified her main reason for smoking: to reduce her anger. She also checked off several other items on the checklists: likes smoking a cigarette with her cup of coffee (lifestyle benefit); helps her relax (another emotional benefit); smokes with her women friends (a relationship benefit); helps her deal with her mother's terminal illness (a coping benefit); helps her concentrate at work (a work-related benefit); likes smoking at parties (a social benefit); and derives a special purpose from smoking in that it helps her connect to a community of other smokers (a spiritual benefit).

In contrast, Mr. B. did not check off any emotional benefits for smoking on first reviewing the list, but did identify smoking as a way to cope with work stress. Only after going through the workbook several times did he begin to realize how much he used smoking to handle his negative feelings. Smoking had acted as a shield against acknowledging such feelings. Mr. B. took several months to fully understand his reasons for smoking. Habitual and addicted smokers may lose touch with why they began and continue to smoke. (For this and other reasons, you may have some difficulties in using the checklists on your first attempt. Whether or not this occurs for you, it does help to look at the options again, as you may have overlooked something.)

Place a check mark (✔) for each benefit that applies to you. If you are like Mrs. G., you will find this exercise easy to do, and you will check off several items. Whatever you check off, you should write down on your decision balance when you do the next exercise. If you are more like Mr. B., you may have difficulty in checking off the items. If so, come back to the checklist later after thinking about it. Or, consider asking someone who knows you to look over your responses to see if that person agrees with you.

Check off any lifestyle benefits that apply to your **unhealthy** habit:

Satisfies likes (e.g., the taste of cigarettes or beer)	
Satisfies needs (e.g., my nicotine addiction)	
Avoids extra costs (e.g., special diets/health clubs)	
Avoids inconvenience to self	
Avoids inconvenience to family	
Avoids disrupting daily routines	
Add any other lifestyle reason:	

Check off any emotional benefits that apply to your **unhealthy** habit:

Increases:		Reduces/avoids feelings of:	
Relaxation		Anxiety and panic	
Expression of anger		Anger	
Self-esteem		Low self-esteem	
Confidence		Inadequacy	
Courage		Fear	
Sexual pleasure		Sexual anxiety	
Intimacy		Loneliness	
Feeling powerful		Powerlessness	
Feeling "high"		Feeling depressed	
Feeling sociable		Anxiety in groups	
Add any other emotional reason:			

Check off any relationship benefits that apply to your **unhealthy** habit:

Helps in making friends	
Deals with difficult relationships/situations	
Avoids difficult relationships/situations	
Avoids personal responsibilities	
Gets back at someone by acting self-destructively	
Add any other relationship reason:	

Check off any coping benefits that apply to your **unhealthy** habit:

Helps in stressful events	
Helps with losses (disability, loss of function)	
Helps with illness in the family	
Helps with death of a family member/friend	
Relieves unresolved grief	
Add any other coping reason:	

Check off any work-related benefits that apply to your **unhealthy** habit:

Helps with work overload	
Helps when unemployed	
Eases job insecurity	
Helps changes in work patterns	
Add any other work-related reason:	

Check off any social benefits that apply to your **unhealthy** habit:

Influenced by:	
Friends	
Family	
Customs	
Work situations	
Add any other social reason:	

Check off any spiritual benefits that apply to your **unhealthy** habit:

Helps cope with a lack of:	
Purpose in life	
Meaning of life	
Life-fulfilling values	
Sense of community	
Connection to a "higher power"	
Add any other spiritual reason:	

Write out a response to this learning exercise and then rate its usefulness in the box below.

1	Use the 0-10 scale to rate how helpful this exercise was to you.	

Please record your score on page 46

2. USE A DECISION BALANCE

Now that you understand some of the forces behind your unhealthy habit, it is time to work on a decision balance. Comparing how Mrs. G. and Mr. B. used a decision balance may help you understand how to fill out your own.

On her first attempt, Mrs. G. listed many reasons to smoke and to quit on her decision balance. It helped her think about her anger in more productive ways. (Ignore what the "think" and "feeling" scores mean for now. The next section will explain.)

Reasons to smoke	Reasons to quit
1. Benefits of smoking *Reduces her anger* *Helps her cope with stress of divorce* *Helps her relax*	**2. Concerns about smoking** *Not using her anger effectively* *Not letting husband ruin her health* *Has shortness of breath*
3. Concerns about quitting *Worst time to quit because of stress from divorce* *Will gain weight* *Nicotine withdrawal symptoms*	**4. Benefits of quitting** *Best time to quit – less likely to relapse when stressed again* *Improves her fitness* *Pride in overcoming nicotine addiction*
Resistance Score *Think score = 2* *Feeling score = 4*	**Motivation Score** *Think score = 10* *Feeling score = 8*

In contrast, Mr. B. listed fewer reasons to smoke and to quit on his first use of the checklists. He studied the exercises in this book and added more reasons as he went along.

Reasons to smoke	Reasons to quit
1. Benefits of smoking *Helps him deal with work stress* *Likes to drink beer and smoke*	**2. Concerns about smoking** *Wife nags him* *Heart attack like his Dad*
3. Concerns about quitting *Fear of failing* *Gets irritable at work and home*	**4. Benefits of quitting** *Saves money* *Better health*
Resistance Score *Think score = 5* *Feeling score = 8*	**Motivation Score** *Think score = 6* *Feeling score = 4*

Add the benefits of your unhealthy behavior from the previous exercise to the following decision balance under question 1: "What are the benefits of staying the same?" Then look at the other three questions and write in your responses to them. The decision balance can help you better understand why you want to stay the same (resistance) and why you want to change (motivation). Whatever your readiness to change, you can use the decision balance for different purposes – to think more deeply about change, to help put a plan into action, or to help prevent relapses after you do change.

Decision Balance

Reasons to stay the same	*Reasons to change*
1. What are the benefits of staying the same?	*2. What concerns do you have about staying the same?*
3. What concerns do you have if you were to change your unhealthy habit?	*4. What are the benefits of changing your unhealthy habit?*
Resistance Score *Think score =* *Feeling score =*	*Motivation Score* *Think score =* *Feeling score =*

Once again, complete the usefulness box below.

2	Use the 0-10 scale to rate how helpful this exercise was to you.	

Please record your score on page 46.

3. ASSESS YOUR RESISTANCE AND MOTIVATION SCORES

Using the 0-10 scale (0 means not important and 10 means very important), Mrs. G. and Mr. B. rated their resistance and motivation scores based on what they thought and felt.

Mrs. G. gave a "think" score of 2 and a "feeling" score of 4 for her reasons to smoke. She gave a "think" score of 10 and a "feeling" score of 8 for her reasons to quit. The process of filling out the decision balance helped her to increase her motivation score.

In contrast, Mr. B. initially gave a resistance score of 5 and a motivation score of 6, based on what he thought. He originally forgot to give himself scores for resistance and motivation based on his feelings, until his wife helped him with this task. She had difficulties in understanding his resistance score of 5 and motivation score of 6 based on what he thought, because she knew how much he enjoyed smoking cigarettes. She said, "I know what you think about your smoking but how would you rate your resistance and motivation scores based on how you feel about your smoking?" Mr. B. immediately changed his resistance score to 8 and motivation to 4. His wife helped him understand how he could think one way (he ought to quit) and feel another (I really enjoy smoking). As he reworked his decision balance and re-read the guidebook over several months, he ultimately gave a "think" score of 1 and a "feeling" score of 3 for his reasons to smoke, and a "think" score of 10 and a "feeling" score of 7 for his reasons to quit.

Now look back at your decision balance. You can use a 0-10 scale (0 = Not important, 5 = Moderately important, 10 = Very important) to rate your resistance and motivation scores, based on what you think and feel. Give an overall score from 0 to 10 for all the reasons that you listed in each column.

Based on what you think:
What score would you give your reasons:
a) to stay the same (left column)?
b) to change (right column)?
Based on what you feel:
What score would you give your reasons:
a) to stay the same (left column)?
b) to change (right column)?

Please put your "think" and "feeling" scores at the bottom of your decision balance. Then put your scores for resistance and your scores for motivation in your progress chart on p. 117, along with the date. Remember to fill in the usefulness box below.
Chapter 4 will help you reduce your resistance score and increase your motivation score over time.

| 3 | Use the 0-10 scale to rate how helpful this exercise was to you. | |

Please record your score on page 46.

4. ASSESS YOUR COMPETING PRIORITIES

Competing priorities affect whether you will try and change. Other priorities in your life may reduce the time and energy that you can devote to change. You can get frustrated if you do not consider these competing priorities before making a change. Let's compare Mrs. G.'s and Mr. B.'s priorities over time.

Mrs. G. was going through a major life event (a divorce) that helped her to change her life priorities in a dramatic way. In contrast, Mr. B. did not give a very high priority to quitting smoking at the beginning, but this gradually increased as he read through the guidebook and began to understand his smoking addiction better.

How would you rate your priority to change at the moment?
Pick any number on the 0-10 scale (0 = None, 5 = Moderately high, 10 = Very high).

My priority score to change my unhealthy habit is: _____.
Please date and put your priority score in your progress chart (p. 117).

What are the priorities in your life that make changing your behavior more difficult?
Write in a response.

_____

_____

_____

| 4 | Use the 0-10 scale to rate how helpful this exercise was to you. | |

Please record your score on page 46.

5. ASSESS YOUR ENERGY TO CHANGE

Life circumstances can make it difficult for you to change. You may really want to change, but lack the energy to do it. First compare Mrs. G.'s and Mr. B.'s energy to change.

Mrs. G. had high energy to change, in part driven by anger generated by her divorce. In contrast, Mr. B. had low energy to change, but this gradually increased over time as he began to realize that smoking caused more stress in his life rather than relieving it.

How would you rate your energy level to change?
Pick any number using the 0-10 scale (0 = None, 5 = Moderately high, 10 = Very high).
My energy score is _____. Please date and put your energy score in your progress chart (p. 117).

Why did you give yourself that score?

_____

_____

What would it take for you to increase your energy score?

_____

_____

_____

| 5 | Use the 0-10 scale to rate how helpful this exercise was to you. | |

Please record your score on page 46.

6. ASSESS YOUR MOTIVES FOR CHANGE

For each behavior, you may have different motives (see list below) for why you may or may not want to change it. Your motives may change over time.

A. Indifference: *"I can't be bothered with changing my behavior."*
B. Externally controlled reasons: *"I am changing because other people want me to."*
C. Internally controlled reasons: *"I should, must, or ought to change."*
D. Freely chosen reasons: *"I'm changing because it is really important to me."*

To help you in this exercise, let's look again at Mrs. G.'s and Mr. B.'s stories and compare their motives.

Mrs. G. gave a 10 for her freely chosen motives and a 0 for all other motives. She wanted to quit for herself and for her health. In contrast, Mr. B. initially gave a score of 10 for externally controlled motives, because his family really wanted him to quit. He gave himself a score of 0 for indifference, a score of 10 for internally controlled motives and only a score of 3 for freely chosen motives. He came to realize that his "shoulds" and "musts" to change were like beating himself up. It made him feel bad for not changing. It did not help him, so he decided to stop that kind of thinking. Instead, he gave himself time and space to really think about what was important to him. With time, this process helped him change his scores markedly in favor of freely chosen motives.

Like Mr. B., more often than not, you may have a blend of controlled (external and internal) and freely chosen motives to change. Rate how each group of motives applies to you in the chart below, using the 0 to 10 scale (0 = not at all and 10 = very much).

Using the 0 to 10 scale, to what extent are you	Score
A. *"Not bothered with changing my behavior."*	
B. *"Changing because my family, partner, or friends want me to."*	
C. *"Changing because I feel that I should, must, or ought to change."*	
D. *"Changing because it is really important to me."*	

Please date and put your scores in your progress chart (p. 117).

A high score for indifference (A) means that you do not care about changing. This can occur for a variety of different reasons: feeling sad, uptight or anxious, drinking too much alcohol, using drugs, or dealing with stressful family, social, or living situations. It helps to understand why you can't be bothered to change. You need to address those issues before trying to change.

The higher the score that you give to freely chosen motives, the more likely you are to change for good. What are your motives to change that are really important to you and your life? For example, "I really want to protect my health," or "I want to be a better role model for my children or grandchildren" are significant reasons. Why did you give yourself the score you did for freely chosen reasons?

Now, write a response to the way you scored the different motives.

_____

_____

What would it take for you to increase the score for your freely chosen reasons?

_____

_____

By now, you should have almost completed your progress chart, and by comparing your earlier scores with your more recent ones, you can assess how much progress you have made in your readiness to change.

6	Use the 0-10 scale to rate how helpful this exercise was to you.	

Please record your score on page 46.

Conclusion

Mrs. G. and Mr. B. each filled out a rating chart (see below) after their first reading and recorded how helpful each exercise was for them.

Mrs. G.'s and Mr. B.'s exercise ratings	Mrs. G.	Mr. B.
1. Making a list of how you benefit from your unhealthy habit	9	4
2. Using the decision balance	10	7
3. Assessing your resistance and motivation scores	8	10
4. Assessing your competing priorities	5	1
5. Assessing your energy to change	3	1
6. Assessing your motives for change	7	2

Overall, Mrs. G. rated these exercises more highly than Mr. B., in part because she was more ready to change. Mrs. G. found exercise 1 much more helpful than Mr. B. did because she could easily identify her benefits for smoking. After further review of the book and making a quit attempt, Mr. B. did the exercises again and found them much more helpful.

Exercises 2 and 3 were rated very helpful by both of them. However, Mr. B. found exercise 3 more helpful than exercise 2, since he found it easier to think in broad terms rather than about specific issues. The reverse was true for Mrs. G.

Mrs. G. found exercise 6 much more helpful than Mr. B. did. This was because, unlike Mr. B., she was more driven to change for her own reasons rather than for external reasons. Both of them rated this exercise much more highly after repeating it, as they came to appreciate better the importance of understanding their motives to change.

Now complete your own rating chart on the following page and try and understand the reasons you gave some exercises higher scores than others.

What Helped You Get Ready for Change?

Use the same scale (0 to 10) to rate the helpfulness of using the exercises over time. The chart will also help you keep track of which exercises you have completed.

Page	How helpful were these learning exercises?	Date	Score	Date	Score	Date	Score
36-38	Making a list of how you benefit from your unhealthy habit						
39	Using the decision balance						
41	Assessing your resistance and motivation scores						
42	Assessing your competing priorities						
42	Assessing your energy to change						
43	Assessing your motives for change						

Make notes about the reasons for your scores, and why your scores changed over time.

_____

_____

_____

_____

_____

46

CHAPTER 4:
TAKE CHARGE OF YOUR HEALTH

In Chapter 3, you completed a number of exercises to help you assess your readiness for change based on your resistance and motivation. In this chapter, you will take charge of your health using the following approaches:

> Address internal factors and
> a) lower your resistance score
> b) increase your motivation score
>
> Address external factors and
> c) overcome barriers to change
> d) increase supports to change.

Resistance (tails) and motivation (heads) are the opposite sides of the same coin. When your resistance is up, your motivation is down, and your health loses. The opposite is also true. If you lower your resistance to change, you will become more motivated to change. If you flip the coin over so that heads are up, your health wins! You may wish to review resistance and motivation (Internal factors) in Section A, pp. 25-27.

Increasing supports and reducing barriers can also help you to change. Barriers and a lack of support can be used as an excuse not to change. However, many people change in spite of not being able to change these external factors. Only you can take responsibility for your health, but it does help to have support from friends and family. You may also wish to review the external factors in Section A, pp. 24-25.

Do as many, or as few, of the following exercises as you like. After writing out a response to an exercise, pick a number from 0 to 10 using the scale below to rate whether the exercise was helpful to you. Remember to record your number in the rating box at the end of the exercise and transfer each score to the chart at the end of this chapter.

0	1	2	3	4	5	6	7	8	9	10
Not helpful					Moderately helpful					Very helpful

A. LOWER YOUR RESISTANCE SCORE

Before attempting to change your behavior, try to understand your views, priorities, and values about change. A better understanding of why you do not want to change will help you think more about the possibility of change. You need to find out which methods can best lower your resistance to change. Here are some methods.

1. Explore Further Why You Do Not Change

After identifying some of your reasons not to change, like Mr. B. in Chapter 3, you may discover there are still "forgotten" or "hidden" reasons. Here are two examples to help you understand better why you may resist change even though you are interested in change or want to avoid complications from your behavior.

An overweight patient overate because it made her feel happy (a known reason). As she thought about it more, she realized that she ate more food when she felt overwhelmed, anxious, or depressed (forgotten reasons). During her therapy for depression, her therapist discovered another reason for her overeating. Her father had used the denial of food as a way to control her "bad" behavior (hidden reason). She now felt that eating food was something in her life that she could control. Once she realized that she used "eating" to cope with "bad" feelings, she was able to moderate her overeating when she was depressed.

An 18-year-old girl was on the birth control pill so she would not get pregnant. She went binge drinking with her friends every 2 weeks or so. Getting drunk was great fun for her and her friends (a known reason). They would enjoy recounting their stories the day after. On some occasions, she would get so drunk that she could not remember having sex with a new partner, or even whether he used a condom. She described those occasions in positive ways and dismissed any concerns about getting AIDS. Her friends would consider her a killjoy if she did not drink as much as they did (a concern about change). She did not recognize that she used alcohol to meet deeper needs: to avoid loneliness, meet new boyfriends, and help her mix with people (hidden reasons).

These examples may help you to rethink and identify some unrecognized benefits that you get from your unhealthy habit. For any positive benefits (having fun with friends), there may be hidden, negative ones (avoiding loneliness). Look back at the list of benefits you completed earlier (pp. 36-38), particularly in dealing with negative emotions.

Can you identify any new unhealthy benefits about your unhealthy habit?

_____

_____

_____

| 1 | Use the 0-10 scale to rate how helpful this exercise was to you. | |

Please record your score on page 66.

2. Assess Your Priorities

Look at the items on the decision balance you filled out on p. 40. List, in order of importance, each of your priorities for changing and not changing.

- What is the most important reason to stay the same (left column)? Put a number 1 by this reason. And what is the next most important? Put a number 2 by this reason. Keep numbering the items in this column until you have finished.
- What is the most important reason to change (right column)? Put a number 1 by this reason. And what is the next most important reason? Put a number 2 by this reason. Keep numbering the items in this column until you have finished.

Compare the following example of how Mr. A. assessed his priorities for continuing to drink. (Chapters 4 and 5 will use the example of Mr. A. throughout to give a feel for how someone can use this guidebook over time.)

Mr. A. liked to drink beer for many reasons. After rating his resistance to change as a 7 and his motivation to change as a 4 on his decision balance, he went over it (see below) to rank his reasons to stay the same and to change separately, from the most important to the least important.

Reasons to drink	Reasons to quit
Benefits of alcohol	_Concerns about alcohol_
Likes taste of beer[4]	Bleeding ulcer[3]
Relaxes me[3]	Alcohol withdrawal[4]
Cope with teenage daughter[5]	
Concerns about quitting	_Benefits of quitting_
Anxiety[1]	Be healthier[1]
Miss drinking friends[2]	Family will be pleased[2]
Resistance Score = 7	**Motivation Score = 4**

Of course, you can change your priorities at any time. Did this exercise help you think more about or even change your priorities about behavior change?

_____

_____

_____

2	Use the 0-10 scale to rate how helpful this exercise was to you.	

Please record your score on page 66.

3. Compare Your Priorities

Compare what you ranked as your most important reason to continue the same habit with what you ranked as your most important reason to change. Again, let's look at Mr. A.

Mr. A. compared his most important reason to drink (anxiety if he quit drinking alcohol) with his most important reason to quit (improved physical health). When he made this comparison, it made him realize that he was sacrificing his physical health for psychological health. He really had not thought about this before. The comparison made him want to improve both his physical and psychological health.

How does comparing your most important reason to change with your most important reason to stay the same make you think and feel about change?

_____

_____

_____

3	Use the 0-10 scale to rate how helpful this exercise was to you.	

Please record your score on page 66.

4. Think How Your Behavior Will Affect Your Health over Time

The following exercise encourages you to think more carefully about how your unhealthy habit has affected your health over a period of time. Mr. A. will again provide an example to help you understand the exercise better.

Five years ago, Mr. A. drank 16-20 cans of beer every week. He liked the taste of beer (a lifestyle choice). Alcohol helped him to relax. After starting a new job, he gradually increased his drinking to more than 25 cans of beer per week with his friends to help unwind after work (an emotional reason). He also quit smoking as he felt shortness of breath when playing basketball twice a week. His fitness level improved. He described his health as excellent.

What was your unhealthy habit like 5 years ago?

_____

_____

_____

What was your health like 5 years ago?

_____

_____

_____

Recently, Mr. A. increased the number of beers a week to more than 30 in response to work stress (a coping reason to drink). He stopped playing basketball with friends because of longer work hours and increased family responsibilities with his daughter (aged 6) and son (aged 5). He also started smoking again because of his work stress. A few months ago, he had chest pains and thought he was having a heart attack. His doctor told him that he had had a panic attack. This event made him realize that he drank beer to cope with anxiety caused by work stress. But he did not change his drinking habits. Four weeks ago, he was admitted to a hospital with a bleeding ulcer. The doctors told him that his drinking and smoking make it more difficult for ulcers to heal. They also told him he had a drinking problem. He disagreed with them because he did not get withdrawal symptoms, like his alcoholic father. But he did not tell the doctors this. He stopped drinking beer for a week, but his friends pressured him to start drinking again (a social reason to drink). He regarded his health as fair. He thought about quitting smoking again. He decided to use this book to work on his smoking habit.

What is your unhealthy habit like now?

_____

_____

_____

What is your health like now?

_____

_____

_____

It scared Mr. A. to think about drinking more beer in the future. He felt that his future health would be poor if he increased his alcohol intake. He did not want to die like his father from a bleeding ulcer. If his health gets worse, his plan is to cut back to what he drank 5 years ago when his health was good.

What do you think your unhealthy habit will be like in 5 to 10 years?

_____

_____

_____

What do you think your health and life will be like in 5 to 10 years if you continue with your unhealthy habit?

_____

_____

_____

What do you think your health will be like in 5 to 10 years if you stop your unhealthy habit?

_____

_____

_____

4	Use the 0-10 scale to rate how helpful this exercise was to you.	

Please record your score on page 66.

5. Clarify Your Personal Choice and Responsibility to Change

In the hospital, Mr. A. felt trapped, as if he had no other choice but to drink. Alcohol had become his only crutch. Alcohol helped him cope but also provided a purpose and gave meaning to his life (spiritual reasons).

To what extent do you feel that you have a choice to change?

_____

_____

_____

Until he went into the hospital, Mr. A. had not really thought about his responsibility for changing his drinking habit. His hospital stay made him think about stopping before his health got worse.

To what extent do you feel that it is your responsibility to decide whether to change or not?

_____

_____

_____

| **5** | Use the 0-10 scale to rate how helpful this exercise was to you. | |

Please record your score on page 66.

6. Make a List of Substitutes for Your Benefits

Mr. A. used alcohol mainly to reduce the anxiety caused by work stress. He made a list of other ways to cope with his anxiety.

Original benefit	A list of substitutes for the benefit
Drink to relax and relieve stress	1. Talk to supervisor at work about reducing work stress 2. Listen to music or read a book 3. Exercise (go for a walk) 4. Chew gum 5. Do gardening

How can you get the benefits of your unhealthy habit in different ways? First, pick the most important benefit of your unhealthy habit. Then make a list of 4 different ways to get this benefit in a healthier way. Do the same with other important benefits. This can reduce the score that you gave to the benefits of your unhealthy habit on your decision balance, and will help you reduce your resistance score.

List a benefit	Make a list of substitutes for your benefit
	1. 2. 3. 4.

If you have difficulty preparing this list, ask for help from someone you can trust.

_____

_____

_____

6	Use the 0-10 scale to rate how helpful this exercise was to you.	

Please record your score on page 66.

7. Change Your Views about Your Reasons to Stay the Same

Think about how you can change your views about staying the same. When you first try to do this, you may not come up with any ideas. If this happens, come back to this exercise at a later time and think about it again.

Mr. A. did not do this learning exercise until after working through this book a third time. Originally, he ranked missing his drinking friends as the second most important reason to drink alcohol. After five months, he decided that this reason was not as important as his need to be alone and relax after work. He thought he could unwind better when alone (without drinking alcohol) instead of when drinking with his friends.

How else can you reduce the importance you gave to the benefits of your unhealthy habit?

_____

_____

_____

How can you reduce the importance you gave to the concerns about change?

_____

_____

_____

| 7 | Use the 0-10 scale to rate how helpful this exercise was to you. | |

Please record your score on page 66.

Conclusion

Once Mr. A. had completed as many exercises as possible, he dated and rated the helpfulness of each exercise for reducing his resistance (see summary below).

Mr. A.'s ratings	Date	Score	Date	Score
1. Explore further why he doesn't change	7/96	2	1/97	6
2. Assess his priorities	7/96	6		
3. Compare his priorities	7/96	7		
4. Think about how his behavior will affect his health over time	7/96	8	1/97	9
5. Clarify his personal choice and responsibility to change	8/96	4	1/97	8
6. Make a list of substitutes for his benefits	8/96	5	1/97	10
7. Change his views about his reasons to stay the same	1/97	7		

On his first attempt, Mr. A. rated exercise 4 (Think About How Your Behavior Will Affect Your Health over Time) as the most helpful. He did not do exercises 5-7 at first. He also had difficulties doing exercise 1 (Explore Further Why You Don't Change).

He was not ready to respond to exercise 5 (Clarify Your Personal Choice and Responsibility) and exercise 6 (Make a List of Substitutes for Your Benefits) until a month later. After finally making a list of substitutions for the benefit of drinking, he did not put any of them into action. It was not until he made a New Year's resolution to cut down on his drinking that he finally rated exercise 7 and rated exercises 5 and 6 very highly. In January 1997, he thought more about why he didn't want to change (exercise 1). He realized he needed to spend more time alone to unwind and to find new ways of finding purpose and meaning in his life.

On first reading this guidebook, Mr. A.'s resistance score went from a 7 to a 6. After his third time of doing some of the learning exercises again, he lowered his resistance score to a 3. He ultimately felt that exercise 6 had the most impact on reducing his resistance score.

Have any of these exercises helped you to lower your original resistance score that you filled in on p. 41? If yes, record your new score in your progress chart in Appendix A with the date. If not, what would it take to decrease it?

_____

_____

_____

_____

What do you think would increase your resistance score? This question can help you anticipate the difficulties of changing and prevent relapses.

_____

_____

_____

_____

B. INCREASE YOUR MOTIVATION SCORE

It helps to find the best ways to increase your motivation score. Here are some ideas.

1. Consider Future Events Happening Now

A future event can be negative or positive.

When Mr. A. thought about having another bleeding ulcer (negative event), he thought he would definitely have to cut down on drinking beer. His wife would also be happy (positive event) if he stopped drinking.

Suppose that your unhealthy habit caused a health problem sometime in the future. Now imagine this problem occurring now. For example, "If you had a heart attack now, do you think that you would quit smoking?" If yes, state why you would quit.

_____

_____

_____

If you would not quit in spite of a health problem, why is this?

_____

_____

_____

Or, imagine that you changed your behavior today and saw an improvement in your health in the future. For example, "Say, over the next year, you lost weight, and discovered that you could walk with less shortness of breath and pain in your knees. Would it be worth trying to change now?" If yes, state why you would change.

_____

_____

_____

If you would not change, why is this?

_____

_____

_____

Think about the quality of your life, both in the short term and long term. Is the short-term benefit of your unhealthy habit more or less important than your long-term health? What would help you decide to change before something goes wrong? Please write a response to these questions.

_____

_____

_____

What would help you decide to change now so that something positive could happen in the future?

_____

_____

_____

| 1 | Use the 0-10 scale to rate how helpful this exercise was to you. | |

Please record your score on page 66.

2. Change Your Values

Your values determine whether you stay the same or develop healthier habits. Many people do not spend a lot of time thinking about values, but thinking about your values is the most important thing you can do to help yourself change. To help you with this learning exercise, think about this question: How would you rank-order the following items in terms of their importance to you? Your priorities may change over time.

What do you value most?	Rank-order your values
Being a good parent	
Being a good provider for your family	
Being a good spouse/partner	
Being a good caretaker for your family	
Doing well at work	
Being healthy	
Being the best at what you like to do	
Being a leader	
Developing your hobbies (sports, singing, etc.)	
Managing stress well	
Add any other items of your choice	
•	
•	
•	
•	
•	

After rank-ordering his values, Mr. A. wrote that his family was more important to him than drinking alcohol with his friends. But he continued to drink in spite of what he wrote. This made him think: either he was not doing what he was saying, or he did not really mean what he wrote. These thoughts made him feel uptight and pushed him to be really honest with himself. He thought about whether he was deceiving himself and his family.

What is more important in your life than your unhealthy behavior (such as smoking)?

_____

_____

_____

What is more important in your life than your health?

_____

_____

_____

Compare the values that you wrote down in response to the two questions above. For example, is your behavior (for example, smoking, alcohol use, and lack of self-care) more important to you than your relationship to your spouse, children, or grandchildren? What is really most important?

_____

_____

_____

| 2 | Use the 0-10 scale to rate how helpful this exercise was to you. | |

Please record your score on page 66.

3. Change Your Views about Your Reasons to Change

Think about how to change your views about the reasons you have given to change your unhealthy habit. When you first try to do this, you may not come up with any ideas. If this happens, come back to it at a later time and think about it again.

Mr. A. did this learning exercise after going through his guidebook for the third time. In addition to his family being pleased, he knew that his family relationships would also improve if he changed his drinking habit. This family reason to change became much more important than before in his decision balance.

How can you increase the importance you gave to the concern about your unhealthy habit?

_____

_____

_____

How can you increase the importance you gave to the benefit about change?

_____

_____

_____

| 3 | Use the 0-10 scale to rate how helpful this exercise was to you. | |

Please record your score on page 66.

4. Look at Your "Excuses" for Not Changing

The word "excuse" is not used to make you feel defensive. It is normal to make excuses for not changing. If you listen to these excuses, it can help you better understand what it will take for you to change. Make a list of all your excuses for not changing. Then beside each excuse, write something that argues against it.

Mr. A. did not do this exercise at first because he thought he would have no problems in cutting down on his drinking. In January 1997, he decided to change his drinking habit. He found that it was more difficult than he first thought, so he decided to complete the exercise.

His initial excuses for not changing were:
   1. "I don't have a drinking problem."
   2. "I can stop drinking anytime that I want to."
   3. "I'm under too much stress now to change."

Next to each excuse (above) he wrote:
   1. "I would have a drinking problem if I can't stop drinking."
   2. "It is better to prevent a drinking problem than to wait until it happens."
   3. "This is the best time to change because if I change, I will be less likely to relapse when I am under stress again."

What are your excuses for not changing?

_____

_____

_____

What are your arguments for change?

_____

_____

_____

| 4 | Use the 0-10 scale to rate how helpful this exercise was to you. | |

Please record your score on page 66.

5. Transfer Motivation toward Changing Your Behavior

Think about how you have tried to do something well in your life, such as taking care of your family, running a 10-kilometer race, or doing an outstanding job at work. You can use the same approach to take better care of your health. For example, some mothers put taking care of their children above their own health. Sometimes, they even neglect taking care of their own health, such as keeping their diabetes under control. In time, their health can deteriorate to a point where ironically it can interfere with the ability of these mothers to be good caretakers.

Mr. A really wanted to do an excellent job at work. He had concerns about losing his job if he became unwell. This exercise made him think that improving his overall health could help him do an excellent job at work. In other words, his health became as important as his job.

Write in your example of what you are motivated to do well at. Then take a look at what you wrote down for the learning exercise about changing your values on p. 59.

_____

_____

_____

Can you take this motivation and use it to take better care of your health?

_____

_____

_____

| 5 | Use the 0-10 scale to rate how helpful this exercise was to you. | |

Please record your score on page 66.

Conclusion

Mr. A. dated and rated the helpfulness of each exercise for increasing his motivation (see summary below).

Mr. A.'s ratings	Date	Score	Date	Score
1. Consider future events happening now	7/96	10		
2. Change his values	7/96	5	1/97	10
3. Change his views about his reason to change	1/97	7		
4. Look at his excuses for not changing	1/97	6		
5. Transfer motivation toward changing his behavior	7/96	7		

Initially, Mr. A. only did exercises 1, 2 and 5. In July 1996, he found exercise 1 the most helpful. When he repeated exercise 2 later on, he increased his score from 5 to 10, because he placed a higher value on his health and his family than on alcohol and his drinking friends. He was really willing to change his drinking habit. He felt exercise 2 had the greatest impact in increasing his motivation score from 4 to 8.

Have any of these exercises helped you increase your original motivation score that you filled out on p. 41? If yes, record your new score in your progress chart in Appendix A with the date. If not, what would take to increase it?

_____

_____

_____

What do you think would decrease your motivation score? This question can help you anticipate the difficulties of changing and prevent relapses.

_____

_____

_____

C. OVERCOME BARRIERS

Barriers are external events that make it difficult for you to change; for example, too much work; transportation difficulties; money problems; temptations to continue your unhealthy behavior; negative influence from family or friends; work pressures; and, school, family, and/or housing problems. Overcoming these barriers can help you achieve your goals for change and improve your health. You may wish to review Overcoming Barriers in Section A, p. 25.

At first, Mr. A. avoided trying to reduce work stress. He feared that his supervisor would not think well of him. The guidebook helped him realize that he had other choices. He decided to look for other jobs just in case things did not work out with his supervisor. He did not want his supervisor to think that he was complaining about his job. He talked to his supervisor about how he could do a better job at work. He also asked him for tips about how to manage work stress more effectively.

What are your barriers to change?

_____

_____

_____

How will you overcome these barriers?

_____

_____

_____

| **C.** | Use the 0-10 scale to rate how helpful this exercise was to you. | |

Please record your score on page 66.

D. INCREASE SUPPORTS

Support may consist of many things:
- the number of people who can help you
- the kinds of support available (money, specific help, family encouragement, community resources, or support groups)
- the felt level of support

Whatever the number of people or kinds of support available, what you feel is probably the most important issue. But you may or may not need support to change. Or you may think that you cannot get the kind of support that you need. This guidebook can help you to get the kind of support that you need from family members or friends. It can also help you give the right kind of support to others in helping them change. You may wish to review Supports in Section A, pp. 24-25.

Mrs. A. was more helpful to Mr. A. after she read this guidebook and saw what her husband had written in it. Mr. A. even accepted her idea about seeing a health professional if he could not change his drinking habit. She left this decision to him. He did not think that this was needed at this time.

What kinds of supports do you need to help you change your unhealthy behavior?

_____

_____

_____

How can you increase your supports to help you change your unhealthy behavior?

_____

_____

_____

D.	Use the 0-10 scale to rate how helpful this exercise was to you.	

Please record your score on page 66.

What Helped You Take Charge of Your Health?

Use the 0 to 10 scale to rate whether these exercises helped you over time. The chart will also help you keep track of which exercises you have completed.

0	1	2	3	4	5	6	7	8	9	10

Not helpful   Moderately helpful   Very helpful

Page	How helpful were these learning exercises?	Date	Score	Date	Score	Date	Score
	A. Lower Your Resistance Score						
48	Explore further why you do not change						
49	Assess your priorities						
50	Compare your priorities						
50	Think how your behavior will affect your health over time						
53	Clarify your personal choice and responsibility to change						
53	Make a list of substitutes for your benefits						
54	Change your views about your reasons to stay the same						
	B. Increase Your Motivation Score						
57	Consider future events happening now						
59	Change your values						
60	Change your views about your reasons to change						
61	Look at your excuses for not changing						
62	Transfer motivation toward changing your behavior						
64	**C. Overcome Barriers**						
65	**D. Increase Supports**						

On the next page, make notes about the reasons for your scores, and why your scores changed over time.

Make notes about the reasons for your scores, and why your scores changed over time.

_____

_____

_____

_____

_____

_____

_____

_____

_____

_____

_____

_____

_____

_____

_____

CHAPTER 5:
MAKE PLANS FOR CHANGE

In this chapter, you will learn how to develop your goals and put a plan for change into action. Your resistance, motivation, competing priorities, and energy level affect what you select as your goals. Before selecting them, overcome any negative self-talk. Then use your strengths and focus on solutions. This approach can help you increase your confidence and ability to change. You can also plan how to deal with relapses.

Do as many of the following exercises as you like. After writing your response to an exercise, pick a number using the 0 to 10 scale below to rate whether the exercise was helpful in planning for change. Again, remember to record your score in the rating box at the end of the exercise and transfer it to the chart at the end of the chapter (p. 89).

0	1	2	3	4	5	6	7	8	9	10
Not helpful					Moderately helpful					Very helpful

1. OVERCOME NEGATIVE SELF-TALK

This exercise helps you to express some of the negative thoughts about change that you might be experiencing. To help you, the experiences of Mr. A. will again be used.

Once Mr. A. tried to cut down on his drinking, he found it much more difficult than he first thought. He listed two kinds of negative self-talk (see below), which he thought might be part of the reason for the difficulty. He then came up with his own ideas for changing this negative self-talk.

Negative Self-talk	*Positive Self-talk*
"I just don't think I can do it."	*"If I keep trying, I will build up my confidence and ability to change in time."*
"I don't feel good about how I have used alcohol in my life."	*"I can rebuild myself a new life."*

Negative self-talk can block you from changing. It defeats you before you begin. What is your negative self-talk? Provide your own examples, and develop your own positive self-talk.

Negative Self-talk	Positive Self-talk

1	Use the 0-10 scale to rate how helpful this exercise was to you.	

Please record your score on page 89.

2. USE YOUR STRENGTHS

Mr. A. identified his strength as his ability to perform very well at work in spite of his work stress, which caused him to drink. Another strength was that he had quit smoking five years ago, although he had started up again, which meant he could use what he had learned from quitting to help him change his drinking habit.

Try to remember what helped you make other successful changes in your life. How can those same strengths help you change your unhealthy habit?

_____

_____

_____

_____

What are your strengths?

_____

_____

_____

_____

How can you use your strengths to increase your confidence and ability to change?

_____

_____

_____

_____

| 2 | Use the 0-10 scale to rate how helpful this exercise was to you. | |

Please record your score on page 89.

3. TAKE A TIME-OUT

Time-outs can help disrupt automatic ways of thinking about your unhealthy habit and help you to change it.

Mr. A. would often go to a bar and drink with friends as a way of unwinding before going home after work. Instead, he thought he could go home and tell his wife that he needed a time-out at home to unwind before having dinner together as a family.

How can you give yourself a time-out to think more deeply about changing your unhealthy habit?

_____

_____

_____

| 3 | Use the 0-10 scale to rate how helpful this exercise was to you. | |

Please record your score on page 89.

4. SUPPOSE A MIRACLE HAPPENED TOMORROW

Try to imagine what your life would be like tomorrow if you changed your unhealthy habit.

Mr. A. tried to imagine himself never drinking alcohol again. He knew his wife would be pleased that his physical health would be much improved if he did quit. Furthermore, his family would appreciate him being around more and being more involved in family life.

What would your life be like if a miracle happened tomorrow?

_____

_____

_____

How do you think your family and friends would respond?

_____

_____

_____

| 4 | Use the 0-10 scale to rate how helpful this exercise was to you. | |

Please record your score on page 89.

5. FIND EXCEPTIONS IN HOW YOU BEHAVE

Think about how you handled a difficult situation (feeling stressed) in a healthy way (for example, taking a walk, chewing gum, listening to music) as opposed to behaving in an unhealthy way (for example, smoking a cigarette, drinking or eating too much).

On some occasions, Mr. A. would not go out drinking with his friends after work. He sometimes felt too tired to mix with his friends and preferred to go home and rest.

Identify an exception and describe why you behaved in a healthy way.

_____

_____

What would help you behave in healthy ways more often?

_____

_____

| 5 | Use the 0-10 scale to rate how helpful this exercise was to you. | |

Please record your score on page 89.

6. BUILD YOUR CONFIDENCE TO CHANGE

Resistance and motivation are different from your confidence to change. You may have the confidence but lack the motivation to change. Or, you may lack the confidence even though you are motivated to change.

You may need specific help to develop certain skills. Some people need to learn self-assertive skills: for example, how to say no to alcohol in social settings. In contrast, you may have the skills to change, but lack the confidence to achieve your goal.

When Mr. A. first went through this guidebook and filled out his progress report, he felt very confident (score = 10) that he could change his drinking behavior. But in January 1997, when he actually decided to change his drinking habit, he felt less confident (score = 4) about whether he could quit drinking for 2-4 weeks.

Now, let's assess your confidence to change. Use the 0 to 10 scale (0 = No confidence, 1= Low confidence, 5 = Moderate confidence, and 10 = Very confident) to rate your level of confidence to change your unhealthy habit = _____.

Please date and put your confidence score in your progress chart on p. 117.

Explain why you gave yourself that score.

_____

_____

_____

If you scored below 10, what would it take to increase your score?

_____

_____

_____

| 6 | Use the 0-10 scale to rate how helpful this exercise was to you. | |

Please record your score on page 89

72

7. INCREASE YOUR ABILITY TO CHANGE

Like confidence, your ability to change is different from your resistance and motivation to change. You may have the ability to change, but lack the motivation or vice versa. Some people may overestimate their ability to change, such as heavy drinkers who say: "I could quit drinking alcohol at any time."

Initially, Mr. A. rated his ability to quit drinking as a 10. But when he actually tried to cut down, he found it much more difficult. He then changed his rating to a 4 after he failed to quit drinking for 4 weeks.

Pick any number using the 0-10 scale (0 = No ability, 5 = Moderate ability, 10 = Very high ability).
What score would you give to your ability to change your unhealthy habit = _____

Please date and put your ability to change score in your progress chart on p. 117.

Briefly explain why you gave yourself that score.

_____

_____

_____

If you scored below 10, what would it take to increase your score?

_____

_____

_____

| 7 | Use the 0-10 scale to rate how helpful this exercise was to you. | |

Please record your score on page 89.

8. UNDERSTAND YOUR ADDICTION

If you use nicotine, alcohol, or other drugs, the following information can help you understand the cycle of addiction that keeps you in your unhealthy habit. Because nicotine is the most common addiction (affecting more than 25% of the population), it is a good example of why it is difficult to change an addictive habit. The description of alcohol use can help you understand how people can develop an addictive habit. To learn more about alcohol addiction and to find out if you are physically or psychologically dependent, refer to Appendix D. For more information about alcohol and other drug problems see Appendix E. Or, go to your library.

A. Nicotine Addiction

The typical smoker absorbs about 1 to 3 milligrams of nicotine per cigarette, totaling 20 to 40 milligrams for each pack per day. Most smokers do not understand the vicious cycle of nicotine addiction. This cycle consists of three parts: the stimulant, wearing-off, and withdrawal effects.

At first, nicotine acts as a stimulant. As the drug effects wear off, smokers begin to feel relaxed. After this feeling of relaxation wears off, however, they get withdrawal symptoms. They feel irritable, anxious, tense, or stressed. Smokers do not realize that those uncomfortable feelings or feelings of stress are often due to nicotine withdrawal. They smoke cigarettes to make those feelings go away. This makes it difficult for smokers to know whether they feel stressed because of the nicotine withdrawal or because of the stress they are under. Nicotine addiction deceives people because it makes them think that smoking is pleasurable, helps them feel relaxed, and relieves stress. In fact, they are treating the stress of the withdrawal symptoms without knowing it. This teaches them to smoke cigarettes to deal with other life stresses.

When people quit smoking completely, they get much stronger withdrawal symptoms: anxiety, inadequate sleep, irritability, impatience, difficulty concentrating, and restlessness. These symptoms last for several weeks after quitting. Quitters also get a physical urge to smoke. They feel that they must replace the drug missing from their body. Quitters may also have psychological cravings to smoke for months or years after recovering from the physical withdrawal symptoms. These cravings may be triggered by situations in which they would commonly smoke, such as drinking in a bar, during stressful events, or when having relationship difficulties.

Cycle of addiction

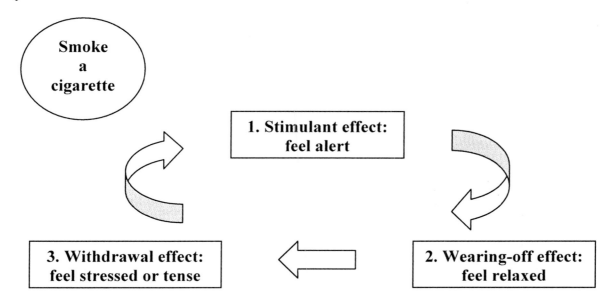

Within the first few days or weeks of quitting, most people start smoking again to stop the withdrawal symptoms. Smokers who have the greatest difficulties in quitting:

- Have had marked withdrawal symptoms on previous quit attempts
- Smoke more than 25 cigarettes a day
- Have difficulties in not smoking in restricted areas
- Smoke more in the morning
- Smoke their first cigarette soon after waking (within 30 minutes)
- Smoke when bedridden with illness
- Inhale more deeply.

Nicotine addiction convinces some people to believe that they have no willpower to quit. Their addiction can seem stronger than their willpower to quit. But smokers can take charge and overcome their addiction. They can now buy the nicotine gum or patch from drugstores to treat their physical addiction. They need at least 50% of their usual amount of nicotine to stop the withdrawal symptoms.

However, quitters face an even greater challenge. They may psychologically crave cigarettes for months, even after the withdrawal symptoms have gone away. Because smokers have programmed their brain into believing that cigarettes help them relax and relieve their stress, their brain will keep reminding them to smoke. People need to maintain their motivation to prevent a relapse.

In what way did the cycle of addiction help you understand more about your unhealthy habit?

_____

_____

_____

Treating nicotine addiction

You can buy nicotine replacement treatments (NRTs) for tobacco addiction from your drugstore. The two types of over-the-counter NRTs are the patch and the gum. The patch more than doubles your chance of quitting. It comes in different doses, depending on which one you select. Treatment usually takes 8 to 12 weeks and may involve stepwise decreases in the dose of nicotine every 2 to 6 weeks. You may experience mild irritation where you wear the patch. Consider taking it off at night if you feel restless and have vivid dreams. Some people still smoke an occasional cigarette while on the patch without relapsing into their usual habit. If needed, you can use the gum for those difficult situations instead of smoking.

While nicotine gum improves your chance of quitting, it is only about half as effective as the patch. However, it is good for people who don't like wearing a patch. The dose from the nicotine gum is 2 or 4 milligrams, with the higher dose being more effective with highly addicted smokers. Half of this dose is absorbed through the mouth. Slowly chew the gum until you notice a tingling feeling or peppery taste in your mouth, and then place the gum between your cheek and gums. After this feeling or taste goes away, you can start chewing again and go through the same cycle. Fast chewing releases too much nicotine and causes side effects. You can chew a piece of gum every 1 to 2 hours for the first 6 weeks, every 2 to 4 hours for the next 3 weeks, and then every 4 to 8 hours for the next 3 weeks.

If you don't like the gum or patch, you can get newer treatments (a nasal spray or an inhaler) from your doctor. The nasal spray method delivers nicotine more quickly than the gum, patch or inhaler, but less rapidly than cigarettes. Quitters can use 1 to 2 doses per hour for up to 3 months. The side effects of irritation in the nose and throat, runny nose, coughing, and watery eyes usually wear off within a week. The inhaler has the advantage of giving quitters a substitute for the hand-to-mouth behavior of smoking. This method is most similar to the gum because the inhaler delivers nicotine into the mouth whether or not you inhale deeply.

If NRTs do not work, you can ask your doctor about a new drug, bupropion (Zyban), to help you quit. Bupropion decreases your urge to smoke. Your doctor can prescribe this drug for treating nicotine addiction. However, if you have a history of seizures, poor appetite, heavy alcohol use or head trauma, you should not use it. This drug can double your chance of quitting. You take a 150-milligram tablet twice a day one week before the quit date and continue for 7 to 12 weeks. If either bupropion (Zyban) or a NRT do not work, it may help to use both of these treatments together.

Mr. A. had quit smoking five years ago but started up a year and a half ago. The most important information that he learned from reading about nicotine addiction was that it could increase his overall stress rather than decrease it. This surprised him because he thought it helped him to relax. This information made him think about whether to quit smoking again.

How does this information help you overcome your nicotine addition?

_____

_____

_____

B. Alcohol Use, Problems, and Dependence

In contrast to nicotine (stimulant), alcohol is a depressant. In other words, whenever you have unpleasant feelings, alcohol can help reduce your feelings of anxiety, panic, tension, stress, anger, low self-esteem, feelings of inadequacy, fear, sexual anxiety, loneliness, powerlessness, depression, and anxiety in group settings. The cycle of alcohol use (see diagram) can help you understand how alcohol can change negative feelings into positive ones in the short term. Thus, people can claim that alcohol helps them to relax, relieve tension and stress, suppress anger, enhance their self-esteem and confidence, give them courage, enhance sexual pleasures and intimacy, and feel powerful, good, high, or sociable, even when the opposite is true.

Cycle of Alcohol Use

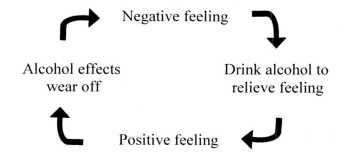

Negative feeling

Alcohol effects
wear off

Drink alcohol to
relieve feeling

Positive feeling

Two examples will clarify how the cycle of alcohol use can deceive people in ways that increase their alcohol use over time. A person may feel depressed and drink alcohol to relieve this feeling. As the short-term benefits of alcohol effects wear off, the depression gets worse and so the person drinks more to relieve the depression.

Alcohol can also help people feel good or "high." Some people may not realize that they use alcohol to overcome their feelings of low self-esteem and low confidence in order to feel good. As the alcohol effects wear off, they don't feel good, so they drink more.

This cycle of alcohol use can help us understand how some people unknowingly go into a downward spiral and start developing alcohol problems and dependence. To help you, a family member, or friends assess whether you or they are developing alcohol problems or dependence, refer to Appendix D for self-assessment.

People may overuse alcohol for other reasons. For example, some people drink alcohol to help them get to sleep. It does help, but it also causes wakeful sleep. People do not realize that they are often getting poor quality sleep. In particular, they do not get enough deep sleep to renew their energy. So, the next day, they feel tired and have difficulty coping with everyday stress. In the evening, they feel stressed out so they drink to get to sleep. It is a vicious cycle. What makes this worse is that their sleeping problem can increase when they stop drinking alcohol because of the rebound effect – restless nights with vivid dreams. It may take a week or so, sometimes much longer, for people to get over how they used alcohol to help them get to sleep.

Mr. A. did not know that alcohol could cause poor quality sleep and make him feel tired. It never occurred to him that if he stopped drinking and slept better, he could have more energy and cope more effectively with work stress. But he was concerned that if he quit drinking, his sleeping problem might get worse before getting better.

How does this information help you understand your alcohol use?

_____

_____

_____

8	Use the 0-10 scale to rate how helpful this exercise was to you.	

Please record your score on page 89.

9. SELECT YOUR GOALS

The goals for change are broken down into three steps based on chapters 3-5. Step 1 (Get ready for change) and step 2 (Take charge of your health) help you change your views and values in ways that give you the motivation to make plans to change your unhealthy habit (step 3). If you still feel the need to get ready for change, work on step 1. If you want to understand further how to take greater charge of your health, work on Step 2. If you want to put your plan for change into action, work on Step 3. Tables are provided for each step to help you select your goals, or make up your own goals. Write them in on the goal chart in Appendix A, and use the scale (0 = None, 10 = Very high) to rate whether you can achieve your goals.

Step 1. Get Ready for Change
Your decision balance (see p. 40) can help you get ready to change your unhealthy habit by helping you understand some of the forces behind change.

On first reading the guidebook, Mr. A. used his decision balance to understand better why he gave himself a resistance score of 7 and a motivation score of only 4, in spite of his health problems.

Here are goals for helping you to think about ways to change your unhealthy habit. Number the three that are most important for you to think about. Date and write them in your goal chart in Appendix A.

Goal Options for Getting Ready to Change	Check
Monitor what decreases or increases my readiness to change	
Think more seriously about the benefits of my unhealthy habit	
Revisit my decision balance and add new items	
Understand better the scores that I put on my decision balance	
Understand better why I want to change	
Understand better what increases and decreases my energy to change	
Understand better what increases and decreases my priority to change	

Step 2. Take Charge of Your Health
Your decision balance can also help you think more about your views and values in ways that help you take charge of your health.

When Mr. A. reread the guidebook, he initially found that thinking about the effects of his drinking habit over time was the most effective way of lowering his resistance score. However, he found that making a list of substitutes for the benefit of drinking alcohol became more effective in reducing his resistance score.

To increase his motivation score, he initially found that the exercise about positive and negative future events occurring now was the most helpful. When he reread the guidebook, the exercise about values challenged him to think the most about change. He realized he was saying one thing (family and health are more important than drinking alcohol), but he was not doing anything about it. This exercise eventually had the greatest impact on increasing his motivation score from 4 to 8.

Select the goals that will help lower your resistance and increase your motivation to change. Which goals will help you the most to take charge of your health? Please date and write them in the goal chart in Appendix A.

Goal Options for Taking Charge of Your Health	Check Any
A. Lower Your Resistance Score Find better ways of substituting the benefits of my unhealthy habit	
Think about how to address my concerns about change	
Learn more about how to overcome nicotine, alcohol, or drug withdrawal	
Understand better my priorities about changing my unhealthy habit	
Think more about what are the most important things in my life	
Think about how I can take more responsibility for improving my health	
B. Increase Your Motivation Score Use the Internet, library, and books to learn more about my unhealthy habit	
Think more about how my unhealthy habit will damage my future health	
Think about changing now if my unhealthy habit has caused a problem	
Think more about how my health will improve if I change my unhealthy habit	
Think about how to overcome my excuses for not changing my unhealthy habit	
Work on how I will change for my own freely chosen reasons	
Transfer motivation from one important activity to changing my unhealthy habit	

You can also take charge of your health if you increase your supports and reduce your barriers to change. Here are some examples of goals that may apply to you.

Examples of Barriers and Supports to Change
Reduce Barriers
Discourage others from nagging you to change
Address transportation difficulties
Overcome money problems
Increase Supports
Tell my family how they can best support my efforts to change
Attend community support groups such as Alcoholics Anonymous, and diabetes resource centers
Seek professional help about treating withdrawal syndromes and addictions

How will you prepare yourself to change within one month?

_____

_____

_____

Step 3. Put a Plan of Change into Action

Pick a date to change within the next week. Your goals could be short term (from a day to several weeks) or long term (from months to years), and pragmatic (10-pound weight loss) or ideal (average weight for height). Even if you do not accept the ideal recommendations for change, you can still work toward reducing your risks and the harm caused by any unhealthy habit. Any small step toward a goal **is better than no change at all.**

In January 1997, Mr. A. tried to cut down on his drinking. He found it much more difficult than anticipated. Instead, his doctor asked him to stop drinking for 2-4 weeks as an experiment to see what he would learn from trying to do this.

Now select or modify any of the goals (see list of options over the page) based on your unhealthy habit. Date and write your goals in the goal chart in Appendix A.

Examples of Goal Options for Taking Action to Change	Check Any
Smoking:	
Cut down my cigarettes by one cigarette each day	
Reduce my smoking by half	
Set a quit date in five days	
Quit smoking again as soon as possible after a relapse	
Alcohol:	
Cut down to low-risk drinking for two weeks	
Abstain from alcohol for two weeks	
Keep to low-risk drinking for the rest of my life	
Abstain from alcohol for the rest of my life	
Weight Issues:	
Stop gaining weight	
Keep my weight the same weight and feel good about myself	
Lose six pounds in six weeks	
Maintain a 20-pound weight loss over two years and longer	
Diet:	
Stick to a 1500-calorie diet	
Follow a low-cholesterol, low-fat American Heart Association diet	
Follow a 2-gram salt diet	
Follow my diabetic diet	
Exercise:	
Exercise 20 minutes, 3 times a week	
Exercise 40 minutes, 3 times a week	
Do rigorous exercise for 40 minutes, 3 times a week	
Do a training program for a 10-kilometer race	

9	Use the 0-10 scale to rate how helpful this exercise was to you.	

Please record your score on page 89.

10. PREVENT RELAPSES

A relapse is when you return completely to your old habit after changing. For example, a smoker makes a quit attempt but within 6 days is back to smoking a pack of cigarettes a day. To prevent relapses, you have to think about how to handle temptations, urges, and cravings. Additional reasons for a relapse are stress, positive and negative feelings, and high-risk situations. After doing this exercise, write out a plan of how you can prevent possible relapses on a separate sheet of paper and put it in your purse or wallet for easy access. This plan can remind you what to do in times of crisis. When you relapse, you may also benefit by working through Chapter 4 so you can maintain your motivation to prevent these relapses.

A. Temptations

Mr. A. felt that his greatest temptation would be after work when his friends would try to persuade him to go drinking. He thought he should explain to his friends that he was medically advised to stop drinking because of the effects of alcohol on his ulcer.

What might tempt you to go back to your unhealthy habit?

_____

_____

_____

How will you deal with those temptations differently?

_____

_____

_____

If your temptations got the better of you in the past, what did you learn about yourself?

_____

_____

_____

B. Physical Urges

For addictive habits, physical urges are part of the withdrawal symptoms that occur in the first couple of weeks after quitting. For example, families may not even realize what alcohol addiction is and may not understand the physical urge to drink.

Mr. A. knew that he was not an "alcoholic" like his father, but would not tolerate anybody telling him what to do about his drinking. His wife tried on many occasions to stop him from drinking because she was worried that he would end up like his father and brother. She could not stop herself from nagging him because she cared for him so much. He resented her nagging and felt more appreciated by her when she stopped nagging.

Mrs. A. read this guidebook and read what her husband had written in Chapters 3 and 4. It helped her to stop nagging him. Instead, she tried to understand better why he liked drinking so much. After reading Chapter 6 (Helping Others), she told him that only he could decide what to do about his drinking habit. She stopped trying to control his behavior. She was surprised how difficult this was for her to do.

She also read the Self-evaluation for Alcohol Dependence (see Appendix E) and thought her husband would give a positive response to at least 10 of the items on the checklist. But she did not tell him what she thought. Instead, she encouraged him to read through Appendix E himself so that he could make sure that he would not end up like his father. After reading the self-evaluation, Mr. A. responded yes to the following questions:

1. Compared to his past, he now spends more time drinking than on exercising with friends.
2. He admits to spending a lot of time getting pleasure from drinking alcohol, particularly when drinking with friends after work and watching football games.
3. He often drinks more than he intends, particularly when his football team wins.
4. He was surprised that he craved drinking beer after stopping for a few days since his last hospitalization.
5. He can drink a six-pack quickly without getting a drunk feeling like he used to.

He was surprised that three or more positive responses to Appendix E could indicate that he was dependent on alcohol. He had difficulty in thinking that he could be on his way to becoming an alcoholic. He thought he could control his drinking if he wanted to. He enjoyed drinking with his friends; it is a guy thing to do.

How will you deal with the physical urge to smoke cigarettes, drink alcohol, or use drugs?

_____

_____

If your urge got the better of you in the past, what did you learn from that experience?

_____

_____

C. Psychological Cravings

Cravings are not due to withdrawal symptoms. They are a result of forming habits. Old habits die hard. You may still crave a return to your old habits long after the physical withdrawal symptoms have gone away.

After leaving the hospital, Mr. A. stopped drinking but had cravings to drink beer. He started drinking again but at a much lower level, about 20 beers a week.

How will you deal with your cravings?

_____

_____

_____

If your cravings got the better of you in the past, what did you learn about how to overcome these cravings?

_____

_____

_____

D. Stress

Mr. A. felt that work stress was his greatest reason for drinking alcohol. He thought he had to work out better ways of reducing and dealing with work stress. In particular, this guidebook helped him decide to speak to his supervisor about his work stress.

What kinds of stress will make you go back to your unhealthy habit?

_____

_____

_____

How can you handle stress in healthy ways?

_____

_____

_____

If stress got the better of you in the past, what did you learn about how to cope with stress in healthy ways?

_____

_____

_____

E. Positive and Negative Feelings

Mr. A. could easily identify bad feelings that could trigger his drinking: for example, anger toward his supervisor and anxiety about whether he could perform well at work. But he had never thought about how good feelings could also trigger his drinking: for example, after watching his football team win.

What positive or negative feelings trigger lapses or relapses?

_____

_____

_____

How can you deal with those feelings in healthy ways?

_____

_____

_____

If your feelings triggered a relapse in the past, what did you learn about how to prevent a relapse?

_____

_____

_____

F. High-risk Situations

Mr. A.'s greatest temptation to drink a lot of alcohol was while watching football games at a friend's house. He drank less when they came to his house. He had two choices: not to go to his friend's house, or to tell his friends that he couldn't drink alcohol or could only have a couple of beers. But he was not sure he could stick to just a couple of beers. This concern changed his choices to being alone and having no friends, or having to make new friends. He thought about whether his friends were real friends or not. Was drinking alcohol more important to his friends than their friendship was to him?

This question really got him thinking about himself. Was drinking alcohol more important than friendships? Or, was his friendship more important than drinking alcohol? He was not sure how to answer these questions; they scared him a little.

Write down high-risk situations that may cause a relapse.

_____

_____

_____

How did you deal with high-risk situations in healthy ways?

_____

_____

_____

What did you learn about how to prevent a relapse?

_____

_____

_____

G. Dealing with Lapses

A lapse is a slip-up, such as eating too much occasionally, or smoking a cigarette while on the nicotine patch. It is important to stop a lapse from becoming a relapse. You can use the same strategies described for relapse prevention to prevent lapses. For example, you can note the time when you had a lapse and what was happening (for example, thoughts, feelings, and the situation).

Since Mrs. A. had read this guidebook, Mr. A knew that she would not nag him. He could tell her if he had a slip-up at any time, and knew she would pick him up from anywhere if he were over the limit for drinking and driving.

How will you prevent lapses?

_____

_____

_____

| 10 | Use the 0-10 scale to rate how helpful this exercise was to you. | |

Please record your score on page 89.

Conclusion

Mr. A. dated and rated the helpfulness of each exercise for putting a plan into action.

Mr. A.'s ratings	Date	Score	Date	Score
1. Overcome negative self-talk	2/97	6		
2. Use your strengths	1/97	4		
3. Take a time-out	1/97	5		
4. Suppose a miracle happened tomorrow	2/97	3		
5. Find exceptions in how you behave	1/97	4		
6. Build your confidence to change	1/97	0	2/97	8
7. Increase your ability to change	1/97	0	2/97	8
8. Understand your addiction	1/97	9		
9. Select your goals	8/96	10	2/97	10
10. Prevent relapses	2/97	9		

Mr. A. rated exercise 9 the most helpful because he liked making the choice about selecting the goals for change, and when. He liked being in charge of himself. He initially rated his confidence and ability to change as 10s on his progress chart and so did not find exercises 6 and 7 as helpful. After failing to quit drinking, he changed his confidence and ability to change ratings to 4 and 3, respectively. He then rated exercises 6 and 7 very highly as they helped him realize that alcohol might be in charge of him. Exercise 8 helped him learn more about how he used alcohol. He also found Appendix D both useful and a little frightening as it made him think more about whether he was really in charge of his alcohol use.

What Helped You Put a Plan into Action?

Use the 0 to 10 scale to rate the helpfulness of using the exercises over time. After rating these 10 exercises, you can assess whether they helped you change any of your scores on the progress chart in Appendix A.

Page	How helpful were these learning exercises?	Date	Score	Date	Score	Date	Score
68	Overcome negative self-talk						
69	Use your strengths						
70	Take a time-out						
70	Suppose a miracle happened tomorrow						
71	Find exceptions in how you behave						
72	Build your confidence to change						
73	Increase your ability to change						
74	Understand your addiction						
79	Select your goals						
83	Prevent relapses						

Make notes about the reasons for your scores, and why your scores changed over time.

_____

_____

_____

_____

_____

_____

_____

_____

_____

_____

_____

_____

_____

_____

_____

SECTION C:
HELPING OTHERS

This section is designed to help you help others who may or may not be thinking about change; in other words, to act as a coach. First, you need to understand the difference between being a controlling versus a motivational coach. Once you are willing to understand that family members and friends may not always follow your advice to change their unhealthy habits, you will learn to stop trying to control their unhealthy habit and move toward motivating them to change themselves (Chapter 6). You'll also learn how to be a preventive coach to children (Chapter 7).

One of the hardest things to learn is that if you persist in advising others to change, they may feel that you are nagging or trying to control them (Coach C). Nagging can make some family members resist change even more, particularly if you try to control them or make change happen. They may get frustrated with you and, in turn, you get frustrated. It can feel like a tug of war. When you pull, so does the other person, but in the opposite direction.

Instead, put down the rope. Try to understand where you both stand on this health issue. You will work more effectively with family and friends if you can learn how to become a motivational coach (Coach M). If you understand better why they do not want to change, you are both more likely to understand your differences in ways that help them think more about change. You can also help them become their own health coach by working through Chapters 3-5 with them. That way, both of you can get a better understanding of how change takes place. Even if they do not change, this approach can reduce your frustration in helping others.

COMPARING A CONTROLLING AND A MOTIVATIONAL COACH

Coach C (controlling)

As Coach C, you care about others and want them to change immediately. You tell them what is wrong or bad about their behavior. You advise them to change ("You've got to lose weight, exercise more, quit smoking, stop drinking, brush your teeth, etc."). In effect, you are trying to control them as you help them change. You also run the risk of imposing your values and views about health on them. If you work in a hurry, you may fail to understand why they see their behavior differently from you. When you select a goal for change, this may lead to conflicts.

Coach M (motivational)

As Coach M, you try to motivate family and friends to change and also to act as a preventive coach to children. You help people understand their choices and the consequences of their actions and still support their right to choose. You may even acknowledge their right not to change, but that does not mean that you agree with them.

You also learn about how your differences in views and values affect how you can work together. Because you try to understand how they view the benefits and concerns about staying the same and changing, they feel as though they have a coach who works with them rather than against them. You encourage them to consider changing their views and values about their behavior. Instead of convincing them to change, you help them think about and select goals for change. In time, they are more likely to change because they really want to, and not just because of what others think. This approach is also more likely to help people take responsibility for the consequences of their actions, whatever their decision.

Comparing Coach C and Coach M

Coach C tries to control others and **directly** confronts them about the risks and harm of their behavior. Coach M uses his or her influence to help others confront themselves about the need for change. The table below summarizes the differences between the two coaches.

Coach C	Coach M
• Assumes too much or too little responsibility for helping others change	• Helps others take responsibility for change
• Controls relationships; tries to make others change	• Fosters supportive relationships; acknowledges others' choice to change or not to change
• Confronts others about their unhealthy habit	• Helps others confront themselves about their unhealthy habit
• Directs others to change	• Explores the issue of change
• Imposes views and values about health and disease on others	• Helps others decide whether to change their views and values about behavior change

As a consequence of working in different ways, Coach C and Coach M achieve different kinds of outcomes in working with others (see table below).

Coach C	Coach M
• Feels frustrated, angry or sad when change does not happen • Argues • Makes family/friends feel as if they ought to change	• Feels good about working together • Discusses • Helps family/friends increase their willpower to change

CHAPTER 6:
BECOME A MOTIVATIONAL COACH

This chapter helps you use your different perspectives on and assumptions about family members and friends to make a difference in healthy ways. Before discussing these differences, it can help to understand:

- How assumptions can help and hinder change
- Why people resist changing their unhealthy habit
- How people resist change

Once you have a clearer picture about these issues, a six-step approach (described beginning on page 99) can help you become a more effective motivational coach. You are then ready to share and discuss goals for change and help family and friends measure their progress over time.

UNDERSTAND HOW ASSUMPTIONS HELP AND HINDER CHANGE

Your assumptions can either help or hinder your efforts to help others change. The following learning exercise may help you identify and think about your assumptions when working with others.

1. Think about a time when a person wanted you to change but you did not want to (and at a later time, you realized, or already knew, that this was the right thing to do).

2. Thinking about the other person, what assumptions did this person make that helped you or made it difficult for you?

3. Thinking about yourself, how did you think this person's effort helped, or did not help, you change?

Now think about what assumptions you are making that help or hinder others from making a change. The following tables can help you think about which assumptions hinder change and which ones help you to help others change. Check off your response to the statements using the scale below.

SA = Strongly Agree, **A** = Agree, **N** = Neutral, **D** = Disagree, **SD** = Strongly Disagree

"Stumbling-block" Assumptions	SA	A	N	D	SD
About yourself • You can make a family member change.					
• You cannot help him think about change.					
About others • He is irrational and does not care about his health.					
• He cannot understand the benefits of his unhealthy habit.					
About your family situation • Family nagging will help him change.					
• Family feels that he cannot change.					

Look at your responses. Do you really believe your answers? For example, you may strongly disagree that you can make others change, but you still try to. In other words, what you think and what you do may be different.

Helpful Assumptions	SA	A	N	D	SD
About yourself • You can tell a family member how you are concerned about her unhealthy habit in nonthreatening ways.					
• You will be more effective in motivating her if you understand how she benefits from this unhealthy habit.					
About others • She is able, but lacks motivation, to change.					
• She is ultimately responsible for change.					
About your family situation • Family can understand why she resists change.					
• Family can help her become her own health coach.					

You may strongly agree with some of these statements, but do you really do what you think you do?

UNDERSTAND WHY PEOPLE RESIST CHANGE

In order to help others change, you must first understand that you may have a different perspective on their unhealthy habit that may hinder you in helping them to change it.

1. Assuming an Unhealthy Habit Is A "Problem"

You may think family and friends see an unhealthy habit the same way that you see it. But, in fact, they may see it as a benefit, pleasure, or solution. The following example highlights how such a habit is viewed both as a solution and as a problem.

Mr. D. enjoyed three beers at night after a hard day's work. It helped him unwind while watching TV. Mr. D. needed time out to relax from his work stresses. In contrast, Mrs. D. felt that his beer drinking was a problem as it took him away from dealing with family responsibilities. She needed his help to put three small children to bed at night.

2. Comparing Views about Benefits

You and your family member or friend may view the benefits of an unhealthy habit differently.

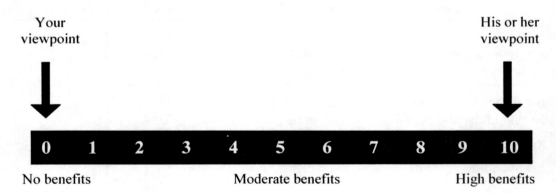

Mr. D. saw his drinking as a way to relax, while Mrs. D. saw it as an unhealthy habit with no benefits to Mr. D. or herself.

3. Comparing Views about Risks and Harms

You and your family member or friend may view the risks and harms of an unhealthy habit differently.

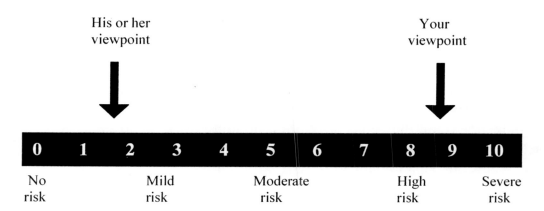

Mr. D. saw no risk in having a few beers because it helped him relax from work-related stress. Mrs. D. felt his drinking was a risk to his health and to the well-being of his family.

4. Jumping Ahead

Because you and others see the benefits, risks, and harms differently, you are at different stages in your readiness to change. You may want them to change even though they are not even thinking about change.

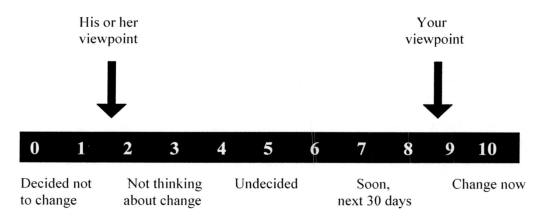

Mr. D. saw no reason to change his unhealthy habit, while Mrs. D. wanted him to change so he could help more with the children.

5. Being Controlling

Have you ever had this experience? Someone threatens your choice to do something, so you hold on to that choice, even when it is not in your best interest. This can help explain why you may cling even more to your choice when others try to control you. You resist the pressure that is put on you.

Mrs. D. kept nagging Mr. D. to quit drinking and help her around the house more. Mr. D. resented the fact that his wife was constantly criticizing him and denied that there was a problem. He refused to think about his drinking or about quitting.

If you act in controlling ways with other people, they are also more likely to resist working with you. People often do not change when being told to, particularly if they feel criticized or judged. Even if they do change, they are more likely to do so because others have instructed them to, or because they feel that they ought to. This approach is less likely to help people change permanently.

UNDERSTAND HOW PEOPLE RESIST CHANGE

Family members and friends may resist working with you in different ways:
- Ignore you
- Avoid you
- Pretend to agree
- Humor you
- Act hopeless about change
- Give up trying to change
- Provide rationalizations about why they cannot change
- Blame you, other people, or their addiction
- Hold others responsible for change
- Deny or minimize that there is a problem
- Rebel against you
- Get angry at you or others

SIX STEPS TO HELPING SOMEONE CHANGE

Using the following six steps can help you to help others take charge of their own health.

Step 1: Use Your Relationship Effectively

You can help family and friends by:

1. Understanding their feelings and views about behavior change
   It is important to understand why they do not want to change, or have difficulties changing. Understanding their feelings and views about their unhealthy habit can help them work on change. The decision balance described in Step 3 can help you all better understand where they are coming from.

2. Clarifying your roles in working together
   You can tell them that you're going to act as Coach M unless they would prefer you to act as Coach C. As a motivational coach, you can clearly state that it is their responsibility to change. You can also use this chapter to help you decide how you can work together in using Chapters 3-5.

3. Relating to them in a flexible way
   To help others dealing with an unhealthy habit, you can relate to them in three different ways: one-up, one-to-one, or one-down.

How You Relate to One Another and Share Responsibility

a. One-up position

Sometimes, it is necessary for you to take the upper hand or the one-up position, particularly when you have to set limits on others who act in inappropriate ways: for example, smoking in your house. You cannot stop them from smoking altogether but you can set limits about what is unacceptable in terms of its effect on you — for example, making them smoke outside. Coach C is more likely to take this position and tell others to change.

b. One-to-one position

Using the one-to-one approach, you work with others on equal terms. You help them achieve their goal for change, but they are responsible for achieving it. You accept that you can't make them change.

c. One-down position

Using the one-down approach, you let others take charge of how to address their unhealthy habits. You may do this in one of two ways.

i) You encourage them to take charge. For example, *"I think you know what you need to do. What would it take for you to think more about changing your behavior?"*

ii) You tell them that you cannot take charge. For example, *"I'm not sure how best to help you think more about changing your behavior. Can you tell me how I can be helpful to you?"*

The one-down position enables you to be very explicit that it is their personal choice and responsibility to decide about whether to think more about change. You give a caring message that you are there to be of any assistance if they would like it, but it is up to them.

Step 2: Decide What to Address

Invite a family member or friend to assess his or her health habits. You can fill out the checklist on the following page while he or she completes the second one. Then compare your views.

Your Assessment of His or Her Health Habits

Circle a letter for each health habit below:
  ***N** = no, not applicable to him/her, not relevant.*
  ***Y** = yes; for each yes response, use the "readiness-to-change" scale:*
       1 = Not thinking about change
       2 = Thinking about change
       3 = Preparing to change

Your assessment of his or her health habits	Response		Readiness to change		
Does not exercise enough	N	Y	1	2	3
Has unhealthy eating habits	N	Y	1	2	3
Is overweight	N	Y	1	2	3
Does not put on his or her car seat belt every time	N	Y	1	2	3
Sometimes forgets to take prescription drugs	N	Y	1	2	3
Does not practice safe sex every time	N	Y	1	2	3
Sometimes forgets to use contraception	N	Y	1	2	3
Uses tobacco products	N	Y	1	2	3

Drinks alcohol more than
    For men: 14 drinks per week
    For women: 7 drinks per week
	N Y
	N Y
			1
			1
				2
				2
					3
					3

Uses illegal drugs	N	Y	1	2	3
Could do more to protect the environment	N	Y	1	2	3
Add your own example	N	Y	1	2	3
How many unhealthy habits does he or she have?					

His or Her Self-assessment of Health Habits

Let your family member or friend fill out the list below.

Circle a letter for each health habit below:
N = no, not applicable to me, not relevant.
Y = yes; for each yes response, use the "readiness-to-change" scale:
    1 = Not thinking about change
    2 = Thinking about change
    3 = Preparing to change

Self-assessment of health habits	Response		Readiness to change		
I do not exercise enough	N	Y	1	2	3
I have unhealthy eating habits	N	Y	1	2	3
I am overweight	N	Y	1	2	3
I do not put on my car seat belt every time	N	Y	1	2	3
I sometimes forget to take prescription drugs	N	Y	1	2	3
I do not practice safe sex every time	N	Y	1	2	3
I sometimes forget to use contraception	N	Y	1	2	3
I use tobacco products	N	Y	1	2	3

I drink alcohol more than
    For men: 14 drinks per week
    For women: 7 drinks per week
	
	N
	N
		
		Y
		Y
			
			1
			1
				
				2
				2
					
					3
					3

I use illegal drugs	N	Y	1	2	3
I could do more to protect the environment	N	Y	1	2	3
Add your own example	N	Y	1	2	3
How many unhealthy habits do you have?					

Then, each of you should make a list of the "yes" responses on the previous two pages and rank them in order of importance. Do this separately before comparing your priorities. This exercise will help you understand what is important for each of you. After, you can discuss your differences, but let him or her decide what to address first.

Step 3: Assess Resistance and Motivation

You, your family members and friends may have very different views and values about change in spite of knowing about the risks and harms of an unhealthy habit. You view the reasons to change (the pros) as being more important than the reasons against change (the cons). However, your family and friends may view their reasons to stay the same as being more important than their reasons to change.

To understand each other better, you both need to assess your differences based on readiness to change, the items you listed on the decision balances, and the level of motivation and resistance to change.

a. Compare Readiness to Change

You and your family member or friend can assess over time whether you are on the same wavelength in addressing behavior change by filling out the exercise below. You can fill this out together or by yourself.

Where are you in trying to help a family member address change? Check below	Readiness to change	Where is your family member in addressing change? Check below
	Not thinking about change	
	Thinking about change	
	Preparing to change	
	Changing behavior	
	Maintaining behavior change	

b. Compare Decision Balances

You and your family member or friend should fill out the following decision balances separately on the next two pages and then show each other what you wrote. After comparing decision balances, you can discuss any differences in the items listed. You can each add new items to your own decision balance, **but only if you want to.**

This exercise can be threatening for some family members and friends. If so, go slowly. For example, complete the decision balance and assess the motivation and resistance scores. Then show each other what you wrote, but do **not** discuss your opinions or differences for at least a day. Use this time to try and understand each other's views better without trying to change one another. Remember, it is important to understand your differences without getting into arguments. Your differences provide opportunities to learn more about each other's views and values.

Fill out this decision balance from your perspective. Wait to fill in the scores at the bottom of this decision balance until you have read the directions for the next exercise on page 107.

Reasons to stay the same (cons)	Reasons to change (pros)
1. *What are his or her benefits from staying the same?*	2. *What concerns do you have about his or her staying the same?*
3. *What concerns would you have if he or she were to change?*	4. *What are the benefits for him or her to change from your point of view?*
Resistance Think score = Feeling score =	**Motivation** Think score = Feeling score =

He or she can fill out a decision balance from his or her perspective. Wait to fill in the scores at the bottom of this decision balance until you have read the directions for the next exercise on page 107.

Reasons to stay the same	Reasons to change
1. What are the benefits for you to stay the same?	2. What concerns do you have about staying the same?
2. What concerns would you have if you were to change?	4. What are the benefits if you were to change?
Resistance Think score = Feeling score =	**Motivation** Think score = Feeling score =

c. Assessing Resistance and Motivation Scores

After comparing your decision balances, each of you should rate resistance and motivation scores from your own perspective, using the scale 0 to 10. Turn to page 41 to remind yourself about how to score resistance and motivation based on what you think and feel.

Turn to page 41 to remind yourself about how to score resistance and motivation based on what you think and feel.

0	1	2	3	4	5	6	7	8	9	10
Not important					Moderately important					Very important

Look at the differences in your scores. Each of you should then write some comments about why you have different views.

Your perspective on the differences:

_____

_____

_____

His or her perspective on the differences:

_____

_____

_____

Then discuss your written responses.

Step 4: Enhance Mutual Understanding

You view and value the benefits and concerns about behavior change differently from your family member or friend. If you do not understand these differences, you will disagree with one another without knowing why.

It is good to discuss your differences on how you view and value the items you listed on the decision balances. Such discussions help to enhance your areas of agreement and address areas of disagreement. You can help family and friends lower their resistance score and increase their motivation score by using the learning exercises in Chapter 4. When their motivation score increases, they are more likely to change.

Step 5: Help Them Achieve Their Goals

After increasing mutual understanding, you can begin to discuss goals for change. These options include:

- thinking more about change
- preparing to change
- taking gradual steps toward change
- taking giant leaps toward change

More examples are described in Chapter 5. You can help family members or friends who are ready for change to develop plans to anticipate how to deal with lapses and relapses.

Step 6: Provide Ongoing Support

You can help others work through Chapters 3 to 5 of this guidebook at a pace that suits them. If they relapse, you can help them learn why they did so, and show them how to use it as an opportunity to start again. The need for your support may vary over time. Either of you may think that it is too much or too little at different times. Discuss what kinds of support and how much support they think they will need over time.

This table helps you understand how the six steps to change assist you in coaching your family member or friend from not thinking about change to not only changing his or her unhealthy habit but maintaining it.

Six steps to help others change	
Step 1: Use your relationship effectively Step 2: Decide what to address first	A. Not thinking about change ➔ Thinking about change
Step 3: Assess their resistance and motivation Step 4: Enhance mutual understanding	B. Thinking about change ➔ Preparing to change
Step 5: Help them achieve their goals	C. Preparing to change ➔ Changing behavior
Step 6: Provide ongoing support	D. Changing behavior ➔ Maintaining change

SHARE AND DISCUSS PROGRESS AND GOALS

If family members and friends allow you, you could read what they wrote in response to the learning exercises in Chapters 3 to 5 of the guidebook. Then you can discuss the scores on their chart at the end of each chapter to identify what is helping them to change. The progress chart they completed (see Appendix A) can also help you discuss whether you agree with the change in their scores over time. It can help in the discussion of why your scores and theirs are different. Such a discussion can help them decide whether to focus on:

- Decreasing their resistance to change
- Increasing their motivation to change
- Increasing their energy to change
- Increasing their priority to change
- Strengthening their freely chosen reasons to change
- Increasing their confidence to change
- Increasing their ability to change

You can also use their goal chart (see Appendix A) to assess whether their goals seem realistic and achievable as they work toward them over time.

CHAPTER 7:
BECOME A PREVENTIVE COACH FOR CHILDREN

There are a number of steps to becoming a preventive coach for your children. First, share your experiences by telling your children how you developed healthy habits and successfully changed unhealthy ones. Even if you have an unhealthy habit, you can still help them learn by sharing information about it. Understand that supports and barriers can also affect whether your children develop healthy habits. Finally, let your children give you their reasons for being tempted to develop an unhealthy habit. It will enable you to work with them to become a more effective coach. Throughout this chapter, smoking will be used as an example of an unhealthy habit because so many kids choose to smoke.

SHARE YOUR EXPERIENCE

If you have used this guidebook, you can share with your children what you have learned about changing your unhealthy habit. You can read chapters to your children so that you can discuss whether they understand how to change. Or, you can let your children read this book themselves and let them ask questions about the exercises and what you have written.

Talking to your children about this guidebook can help them get off to a healthy start. You can help your children avoid developing unhealthy habits. This book shows you how to become a preventive coach to help your children stay on the right track or to help them get back on track if they slip. If you are a smoker or ex-smoker, you can help your children understand nicotine addiction even better, by telling them about your childhood experience with cigarettes.

LEARN ABOUT NICOTINE ADDICTION

In spite of what we know about healthy living, take note of this fact. Tobacco use will cause the greatest worldwide risk for disability and death by the year 2020. Nicotine addiction is the greatest health threat to future generations.

Tobacco companies lied to the government by stating under oath that they thought nicotine was not addictive, when they knew that it was. They also denied direct marketing of cigarettes to children. Parents need to learn more about nicotine addiction so that they can teach their children.

Read the section on nicotine addiction on pp. 74-77 in Chapter 5 to your children. Or, let them read the section alone. Let your son or daughter ask questions about what he or she did not understand. Help them understand what nicotine addiction is all about.

Research shows that most teenage smokers think that they can quit at any time. The fact is that most teenagers become addicted to nicotine five years later. They regret that they ever started smoking. This is the reason why it is important to educate kids as soon as possible about nicotine addiction and the temptation to smoke.

As your children grow up, they also need to understand what will tempt them or pressure them to smoke. They need to know how to say no if they want to. They need to be motivated to say no when faced with peer pressure. Let them ask questions and see whether they have faced a similar or different situation to you.

SUPPORTS AND BARRIERS

Teenagers who have parents and peers who smoke are much more likely to smoke than teenagers who have nonsmoking parents and friends. In the United States, access to alcohol and marijuana at home also increases childhood use. Students who worked in a job more than 20 hours a week used cigarettes, alcohol, and marijuana more than students who did not. Students (aged 16-18) who appeared older than their peers had higher rates of drug, alcohol, and tobacco use and experienced sexual intercourse at an earlier age. Finally, families whose members are critical of each other are more likely to develop unhealthy habits. Thus, family and school factors affect whether children avoid or develop unhealthy habits such as smoking. Understanding how such external events can make change more difficult for your children is an important step to eliminating barriers to change.

Supportive parent-child and child-school relationships can protect your children from developing an unhealthy habit. By increasing such supports, you can help your children prevent or change an unhealthy habit. To read more about barriers and supports, see Chapter 2.

The following exercise will help your child better understand some of the temptations of an unhealthy habit. Fill in the decision balance and share your childhood experience of being tempted to smoke. Rate your reasons to smoke and not to smoke using the 0-10 scale. Discuss your responses with your child.

Decision Balance

A Decision Balance: To try or not to try a cigarette	
1. Benefits of trying a cigarette *"As a kid, what tempted you to consider smoking?" (For example, be a daredevil.)* *"If you smoked a cigarette, what were the benefits of smoking?"*	2. Concerns about trying a cigarette *"When you were a kid, did you have any concerns about smoking cigarettes?" (For example, didn't like the idea of inhaling smoke into your lungs.)*
3. Concerns about not smoking a cigarette *"At any time when growing up, did you have any concerns about never smoking a cigarette?" (For example, get rejected by friends for not smoking.)*	4. Benefits of not smoking a cigarette *"As a kid, did you think about the benefits of never smoking a cigarette?" (For example, stay fit and run faster.)*
Reasons to try a cigarette	**Reasons to never smoke**

UNDERSTANDING YOUR CHILDREN'S TEMPTATIONS

Children face temptation just like adults do. They are taught that the reasons not to smoke, for example, are more important than the reasons to smoke. But as they grow up, they may change their reasons for either trying a cigarette or never smoking one. If the reasons to smoke become more important than the reasons not to smoke, they may be tempted.

As a parent, you can try and understand how your children view the temptations to smoke. You and your child can use the next two pages to compare your views on the temptations. Furthermore, you can repeat these exercises over time to see how your child's views on smoking change as he or she grows up. For example, when children are younger, they may list different reasons than as they get older. Or, they may give a score of 10 for the reasons to never smoke and a zero score for the reasons to smoke in their decision balance when they are 10 years old, but change them as they grow up.

YOUR CHILD'S VIEW

Reasons to try a cigarette	Reasons never to smoke
What tempts you to smoke a cigarette? What are benefits or good things about smoking? **A.** Not letting your friends down **B.** Fitting in with friends **C.** Being cool **D.** Being popular **E.** Seeing what it is like **F.** Relaxing **G.** Movies, TV shows, and ads make smoking look attractive **H.** Smoking with family **I.** Coping with stress **J.** Believing I can try smoking and quit before getting addicted **Top 3 reasons to try a cigarette** #1 Reason: _____ #2 Reason: _____ #3 Reason: _____	***What concerns you most about smoking a cigarette?*** **A.** Scared of smoking **B.** Bad for your health in the long run **C.** Getting addicted **D.** Getting in trouble with parents, teachers, etc. **E.** Smelly clothes and yellow teeth **F.** Losing friends or having bad friends who smoke **G.** Not being able to play sports well or run as fast **H.** Having to go to special places to smoke **I.** Wasting money on buying cigarettes **J.** Dying earlier **Top 3 reasons to never smoke** #1 Reason:_____ #2 Reason: _____ #3 Reason: _____
What concerns you most about NEVER smoking? **A.** Losing friends **B.** Getting picked on for not smoking **C.** Not fitting in **D.** Not being cool **E.** If my friends keep offering a cigarette, I would have to keep saying no **F.** Just wanting to know what it is like **G.** Not looking grown up **H.** Being tempted to smoke all the time **I.** Not being popular **Top 3 concerns about never smoking** #1 Reason: _____ #2 Reason: _____ #3 Reason: _____	***What are the benefits or the good things for you about NEVER smoking?*** **A.** Living longer **B.** Having a healthier life **C.** Not getting addicted **D.** Not getting in trouble with parents **E.** Being proud to be a nonsmoker **F.** Better appearance and smelling better **G.** Having better friends **H.** Being better at sports, running faster, being more athletic **I.** Would not have to cover up smoking **J.** Saving money **K.** Proving I am strong enough to resist smoking **L.** Being my own boss **Top 3 benefits to never smoke** #1 Reason: _____ #2 Reason: _____ #3 Reason: _____

114

YOUR VIEWPOINT

Reasons to try a cigarette	Reasons never to smoke
What tempts children to smoke a cigarette? What are benefits or good things about smoking? A. Not letting their friends down B. Fitting in with friends C. Being cool D. Being popular E. Seeing what it is like F. Relaxing G. Movies, TV shows, and ads make smoking look attractive H. Smoking with family I. Coping with stress J. Believing they can try smoking and quit before getting addicted **Top 3 reasons to try a cigarette** #1 Reason: _____ #2 Reason: _____ #3 Reason: _____	***What concerns children most about smoking a cigarette?*** A. Scared of smoking B. Bad for their health in the long run C. Getting addicted D. Getting in trouble with parents, teachers, etc. E. Smelly clothes and yellow teeth F. Losing friends or having bad friends who smoke G. Not being able to play sports well or run as fast H. Having to go to special places to smoke I. Wasting money on buying cigarettes J. Dying earlier **Top 3 reasons to never smoke** #1 Reason:_____ #2 Reason: _____ #3 Reason: _____
What concerns children most about NEVER smoking? A. Losing friends B. Getting picked on for not smoking C. Not fitting in D. Not being cool E. If their friends keep offering a cigarette, they would have to keep saying no F. Just wanting to know what it is like G. Not looking grown up H. Being tempted to smoke all the time I. Not being popular **Top 3 concerns about never smoking** #1 Reason: _____ #2 Reason: _____ #3 Reason: _____	***What are the benefits or the good things for children about NEVER smoking?*** A. Living longer B. Having a healthier life C. Not getting addicted D. Not getting in trouble with parents E. Pride in being a nonsmoker F. Better appearance and smelling better G. Having better friends H. Being better at sports, running faster, being more athletic I. Would not have to cover up smoking J. Saving money K. Proving they are strong enough to resist smoking L. Being their own boss **Top 3 benefits to never smoke** #1 Reason: _____ #2 Reason: _____ #3 Reason: _____

HELPING CHILDREN RESIST UNHEALTHY HABITS

Becoming a preventive coach will help your children get off to a healthy start. If they ever need to use this guidebook, the decision balance can help children better understand what can tempt them to develop unhealthy habits. If they do develop an unhealthy habit, your experience in using this book may also help them use it effectively to change their unhealthy habit.

APPENDIX A: YOUR PROGRESS CHART

0	1	2	3	4	5	6	7	8	9	10
None				Moderately High						Very High

Monitoring your progress scores over time

Page	Items	Date	Score	Date	Score	Date	Score	Date	Score
41	Your reasons to stay the same (resistance) based on what you think								
41	Your reasons to stay the same (resistance) based on what you feel								
41	Your reasons to change (motivation) based on what you think								
41	Your reasons to change (motivation) based on what you feel								
42	Your overall level of priority given to changing your behavior								
42	Your level of energy that you can devote toward changing								
	Your motives to change:								
44	Indifference – "I can't be bothered with changing my behavior."								
44	Externally controlled reasons – "I am changing only because my family, partner, or friends want me to."								
44	Internally controlled reasons – "I should, must, or ought to change."								
44	Freely chosen reasons – "I am changing because it is really important to me."								
72	Your confidence to change								
73	Your ability to change								

117

APPENDIX A: YOUR GOAL CHART

Date for change	Describe your goals for change	Assess whether you think you can achieve your goal (using the 0-10 scale)

APPENDIX B: EVALUATING WEB SITES

These organizations help to evaluate the quality of Web sites:

1. Discern

http://www.discern.org.uk Originally developed to evaluate consumer health print materials, Discern contains a brief questionnaire that allows the user to assess the quality of a health information Web site.

2. Evaluating Web Resources

http://www2.widener.edu/Wolfgram-Memorial-Library/webeval.htm This Widener University site contains short informational pages that can be duplicated as handouts as long as the Widener logo remains on the sheet. It also has a PowerPoint presentation and other educational resources.

3. Health On the Net

http://www.hon.ch/HONcode/ The Health On the Net Code of Conduct has been written with the Web developer in mind. If the developer follows HON's criteria, they may apply to receive HON's "active seal" icon. A click on the seal takes the user to HON where the criteria are stated and a list of HON-rated quality health sites is available. HON also contains a medical search engine and a variety of other resources.

4. Health Summit Working Group

http://hitiweb.mitretek.org/hswg/ Mitretek Systems sponsors the Health Summit Working Group, whose participants include representatives of the general public, as well as health care providers, medical librarians and related information resources professionals, and Web site developers affiliated with numerous organizations in the health care and information communities.

5. Healthfinder

http://www.healthfinder.gov/smartchoices/onlineinfo/evaluate.htm This one page of the much larger federally sponsored healthfinder consumer information site provides links to a variety of evaluation materials and organizations.

6. Mental Health Net

http://mentalhelp.net/help/ratings.htm Mental Health Net provides evaluation criteria and a four-star rating system for the sites included in its list of links.

7. Nutrition Navigator

http://navigator.tufts.edu/ratings.html This Tufts University site contains a rating guide to nutrition sites, listing hundreds of rated sites.

8. OMNI Advisory Group for Evaluation Criteria

http://omni.ac.uk/agec/ The Advisory Group has studied the emerging issues concerning Web site quality, and reviewed the services of other Web evaluation organizations. The group's overall aim has been "to establish the effectiveness of such services in facilitating access to quality materials available via the Internet."

HEALTH FRAUD AND QUACKERY

Included here are two Web sites that provide a public service to those wishing to evaluate alternative or complementary medicine claims. **The National Council for Reliable Health Information** at http://www.ncrhi.org, and **Quackwatch,** operated by Stephen Barrett, M.D., at http://www.quackwatch.com/index.html offer evidence-driven information about health fraud and quackery appearing on the Internet.

Resources for Evaluating the Web Site Yourself
Vidmar, D. (1999). *Evaluation: What Is a Good Site?*
Available: http://www.sou.edu/library/dale/evaluate.htm
Internet Resource Evaluation: http://www.lib.umich.edu/megasite/bibl.html

Some Recommended Sites

American Council on Exercise
PO Box 910449
San Diego, CA 92191
800-825-3636
www.acefitness.org

American Diabetes Association
1660 Duke Street
Alexandria, VA 22314
800-ADA-DISC, ext. 363
http://www.diabetes.org

American Dietetic Association
216 W. Jackson Blvd.
Chicago, IL 60606-6995
312-899-0040
800-366-1655 consumer nutrition hotline
www.eatright.org

American Heart Association
http://www.americanheart.org

American Lung Association
1740 Broadway
New York, NY 10019-4374
800-586-4872
www.lungusa.org

Asthma and Allergy Foundation of America
1125 15th St. NW
Suite 502
Washington, DC 20005
800-7-ASTHMA
http://www.aafa.org

Center for Health Promotion and Education
Centers for Disease Control
1600 Clifton Road NE
Atlanta, GA 30333
404-639-3311
http://www.cdc.gov

National Council of Patient Information and
Education
666 11th St. NW
Suite 810
Washington, DC 20001
202-347-6711
http://nhic-nt.health.org

National Institute of Mental Health
5600 Fishers Lane, Room 7C-02
Rockville, MD 20857
301-443-4513
www.nimh.nih.gov

National Mental Health Association
1021 Prince Street
Alexandria, VA 22134-2971
800-969-NMHA
www. nmha.org

Shape Up America!
6707 Democracy Blvd., Suite 306
Bethesda, MD 20817
301-493-5368
www.shapeup.org

APPENDIX C: LOW-RISK DRINKING RECOMMENDATIONS

Maximum Alcohol Consumption Per Week

Alcohol	Canada		United States		England	
	Men	Women	Men	Women	Men	Women
Standard number of drinks	12	12	14	7	28	21
Grams per drink	10	10	12	12	8	8
Total grams per week	120	120	168	84	224	168

APPENDIX D: ALCOHOL ABUSE

Self-evaluation for Alcohol Problems

Have you had one or more of the following problems caused by or made worse by alcohol use during the past year?

1. *Difficulties in fulfilling your responsibilities at work, school, or home* .
2. *Physical or mental health problems*
3. *Repeated alcohol-related legal problems*
4. *Social or relationship problems*

APPENDIX E: ALCOHOL DEPENDENCY

Use the code to respond: Y= Yes   Ns = Not sure   N = No

Self-evaluation for Alcohol Dependence	Circle One		
Do less of other activities (social, occupational, or recreational) because of being more involved in drinking-related activities	Y	Ns	N
Spend more time obtaining alcohol and recovering from its effects	Y	Ns	N
Spend a fair amount of time in obtaining alcohol for your pleasure	Y	Ns	N
Spend a fair amount of time recovering from the effects of alcohol	Y	Ns	N
Less able to control alcohol use	Y	Ns	N
Have difficulty deciding when to stop drinking alcohol	Y	Ns	N
Drink larger amounts of alcohol than intended	Y	Ns	N
Have urges or cravings for alcohol	Y	Ns	N
Drink even though it causes problems	Y	Ns	N
Develop or lose tolerance of alcohol	Y	Ns	N
Need to drink more alcohol to have the same effect	Y	Ns	N
Need to drink much more alcohol to get drunk	Y	Ns	N
Need to drink much less alcohol to have the same effect or to get drunk	Y	Ns	N
Get withdrawal symptoms after quitting alcohol	Y	Ns	N
Drink alcohol to relieve withdrawal symptoms	Y	Ns	N

If you responded "yes" to a question from three or more items listed above, you are probably physically or psychologically dependent on alcohol.

APPENDIX F:
ADDITIONAL RESOURCES FOR ALCOHOL AND DRUG PROBLEMS

Telephone numbers

If you think that you may have an alcohol or drug problem, call the National Council on Alcoholism and Drug Dependency Hopeline (1-800-NCA-CALL) or try calling 1-800-662-4357.

If you are worried about a family member or friend who drinks too much, you can get help from calling Al-Anon/Alateen (1-800-356-9996).

If you have a cocaine problem, call Cocaine Anonymous National Referral Line (1-800-347-8998) for help.

Web sites for more information about drugs

Marijuana Anonymous: www.marijuana-anonymous.org/
Cocaine Anonymous World Services: www.ca.org/
Narcotics Anonymous: www.wsoinc.com
Comprehensive Addiction Programs Inc.: www.helpfinders.com